THE HANDBOOK OF RED FLAGS IN MEDICINE

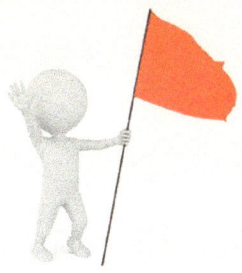

Dr Amir Ahmad FRCP FRCPE FACP
Dr Pooja Sheemar MBBS
Dr Philip Tamang MBBS
Dr Asif Ahmad FRCA

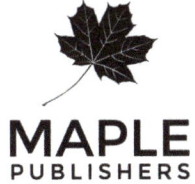

MAPLE PUBLISHERS

THE HANDBOOK OF RED FLAGS IN MEDICINE

Authors: ➡ Dr Amir Ahmad FRCP
➡ Dr Pooja Sheemar MBBS
➡ Dr Philip Tamang MBBS
➡ Dr Asif Ahmad FRCA

Copyright © 2025 Dr Amir Ahmad

First Published in 2025
Second Edition in 2026

ISBN 978-1-83538-513-5 (Paperback)

Published by:
Maple Publishers
Fairbourne Drive, Atterbury,
Milton Keynes,
MK10 9RG, UK
www.maplepublishers.com

The right of Dr Amir Ahmad to be identified as author of this work has been asserted by the author in accordance with section 77 and 78 of the Copyright, Designs and Patents Act 1988.

A CIP catalogue record for this title is available from the British Library.

All rights reserved. No part of this book may be reproduced or translated in any form or by any means, electronic or mechanical, including photocopying, recording or by any information storage and retrieval system without written permission from the author.

The views expressed in this work are solely those of the author and do not necessarily reflect the publisher's opinions, and the publisher, as a result of this, disclaims any responsibility for them.

Preface

Identifying life-threatening and serious diseases is crucial for patient safety. This red book offers a quick review of clinical medicine red flags. I hope readers find it helpful.

Recognising the early warning signs—often called "red flags"—is an essential skill for healthcare professionals in order to make timely diagnoses and initiate appropriate interventions. This resource is designed not only for clinicians but also for students and trainees who wish to strengthen their ability to detect urgent or emergent conditions. The concise summaries and practical checklists included in this book aim to support daily clinical decision-making, enhance patient outcomes, and reinforce safe medical practice. By arming readers with up-to-date information and highlighting critical presentations, the book aspires to serve as a rapid reference both in acute care settings and routine clinical encounters.

Dr Amir Ahmad, Consultant Physician, UK

Dr Pooja Sheemar, Resident Doctor, UK

Dr Philip Tamang, Resident Doctor, UK

Dr Asif Ahmad, Consultant Anesthetist, Dubai

CONTENTS

- Abdominal Pain 5
- Back pain 16
- Chest Pain 26
- Constipation 36
- Cough 46
- Confusion 55
- Diarrhea 64
- Diplopia 75
- Dizziness / Vertigo 85
- Dyspepsia 95
- Dysphagia 103
- Dyspnoea 112
- Dysuria 122
- Edema 131
- Fever 141
- Falls 150
- Gastrointestinal bleeding 160
- Headache 172
- Haematuria 181
- Hemoptysis 194
- Jaundice 205
- Joint Pains 215
- Nausea and Vomiting 225
- Palpitations 235
- Syncope 246
- Tremor 261
- Vision loss 272
- Weakness 287

Abdominal Pain

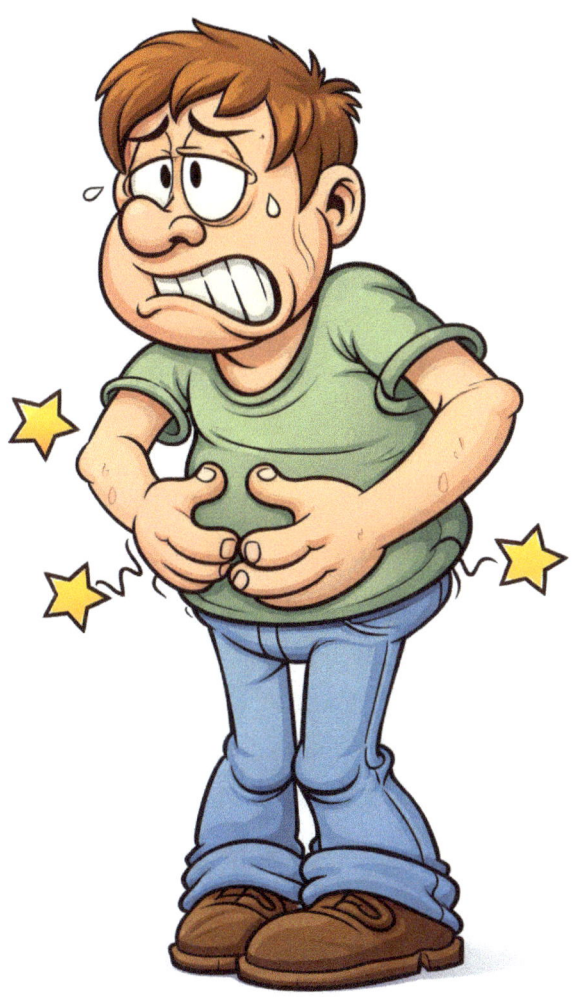

Red Flags: Abdominal Pain

- Abdominal distension/Unexplained vomiting
- Unexplained PV bleed
- Abdominal pain on exertion
- Change in bowel habits
- Unwell diabetic patient
- Severe sudden onset ("acute abdomen")
- Abdominal pain with hemodynamic instability (shock)
- Peritonism (rigidity, rebound, guarding)
- Pain out of proportion to physical findings
- Persistent vomiting (especially bilious/feculent with distension)
- GI bleeding (Haematemesis, Melena, PR bleed)
- Unexplained weight loss/anorexia
- Jaundice with abdominal pain
- Fever with abdominal pain
- Palpable abdominal mass
- Abdominal pain in pregnancy
- Abdominal pain + chest/back radiation
- Elderly patient with severe pain
- Immunosuppressed patient with abdominal pain

∏ Abdominal distension/ unexplained vomiting:
- **Implications/Diagnoses:** Constipation, Bowel obstruction.
- **Investigations:** AXR, PR examination to check Faecal loading/impaction.
- Red Flags

∏ Unexplained PV bleed:
- **Implications/Diagnoses:** Genitourinary Cancer, infections.
- **Investigations:** High vaginal swabs for Chlamydia/Gonorrhea, TV USS. Refer to Gynecology.

∏ Abdominal pain on exertion:
- **Implications/Diagnoses:** Cardiac ischaemia.
- **Investigations:** Troponin and ECG to rule out acute MI
- If negative, Refer to Cardiology for Stress test.

∏ Change in Bowel Habits:
- **Implications/Diagnoses:** Colorectal cancer.
- **Investigations:** urgent CT Abdomen/Pelvis, PR to look for bleeding, Faecal occult blood.

∏ Unwell Diabetic patient:
- **Implications/Diagnoses:** DKA.
- **Investigations:** check Ketones, Glucose, VBG.
- Continue the long-acting insulin always and follow DKA guidelines.

∏ Raised Amylase/Lipase:
- **Implications/Diagnoses:** Pancreatitis.
- **Investigations:** FBC, Serum Lipase/ Amylase and refer to Surgeons.
- Upper abdominal pain radiating to back.

∏ Severe sudden onset pain:
- **Implications/Diagnoses:** Perforated viscus, ruptured AAA, mesenteric ischemia, ruptured ectopic pregnancy.
- **Investigations:** Urgent CT abdomen/Pelvis, Ultrasound abdomen (AAA, ectopic), serum lactate, β- hCG, Bloods.

∏ Abdominal pain with hemodynamic instability (shock):
- **Implications/Diagnoses:** Ruptured AAA, perforation. Massive GI bleed, splenic rupture, ectopic pregnancy.
- **Investigations:** Ultrasound abdomen (FAST), CT angiogram, CT abdomen & pelvis, FBC, Hb, crossmatch, coagulation profile.

∏ Peritonism (rigidity, rebound tenderness, guarding):
- **Implications/Diagnoses:** Perforation, Peritonitis, ischaemic bowel.
- **Investigations:** Erect CXR (free air), Urgent CT abdomen, Blood cultures, Serum Lactate.

∏ Pain out of proportion to findings:
- **Implications/Diagnoses:** Mesenteric Ischemia.
- **Investigations:** Serum lactate, CT mesenteric angiogram.

∏ Persistent vomiting (especially bilious with distension):
- **Implications /Diagnoses:** small/large bowel obstruction, Volvulus.
- **Investigations:** AXR, CT abdomen with contrast, U&E.

∏ GI bleeding (hematemesis, Melanesia, PR bleed):
- **Implications/Diagnoses:** Peptic ulcer bleed, diverticular bleed, IBD, ischaemic colitis, bowel cancer.
- **Investigations:** OGD, colonoscopy, CT angiography, FBC, crossmatch.

Unexplained weight loss/anorexia:
- **Implications/Diagnoses:** GI malignancy (stomach, pancreas, colon), TB, Lymphoma.
- **Investigations:** CT TAP, endoscopy, colonoscopy, tumor markers.

Jaundice with abdominal pain:
- **Implications/Diagnoses:** Cholangitis, Choledocholithiasis, Pancreatic cancer.
- **Investigations:** LFT, USS abdomen, MRCP, CT pancreas.

Fever with abdominal pain:
- **Implications/Diagnoses:** Appendicitis, diverticulitis, cholecystitis, cholangitis, perforation.
- **Investigations:** FBC, CRP, blood cultures, CT abdomen, USS abdomen.

Palpable abdominal mass:
- **Implications/Diagnoses:** Malignancy, AAA, abscess, hepatosplenomegaly.
- **Investigations:** USS, CT abdomen, tumour markers.

Abdominal pain in Pregnancy:
- **Implications/Diagnoses:** Ectopic pregnancy, placental abruption, ovarian torsion.
- **Investigations:** β-hCG, urgent pelvic USS, CT abdomen/pelvis, FBC, crossmatch.

Abdominal pain + chest/back radiation:
- **Implications/Diagnoses:** MI, Aortic dissection, AAA rupture, Pancreatitis.
- **Investigations:** ECG, Troponin, CXR, CT angiogram, amylase/lipase.

∏ Elderly patient with severe pain:

- **Implications/Diagnoses:** AAA rupture, Bowel ischaemia, Perforation, Cancer.
- **Investigations:** CT angiogram, USS abdomen, urgent CT abdomen.

∏ Immunosuppressed patient with abdominal pain:

- **Implications/Diagnoses:** CMV colitis, TB, Neutropenic enterocolitis, abscess.
- **Investigations:** CT abdomen, stool cultures, colonoscopy, cultures.

🔑 Key Points

- Think life-threatening first – AAA, Ischaemia, perforation, ruptured ectopic pregnancy.
- Red flags = urgent referral + imaging + labs.
- Rule out pregnancy in childbearing age women.
- Always in history and exams look for signs of peritonitis, shock and obstruction.
- Acute and severe abdominal pain, however, is almost a symptom of intra-abdominal cause.
- AXR and erect CXR are useful for obstruction, perforation and constipation only.
- USS is useful for suspected biliary tract disease or ectopic pregnancy (transvaginal), can also detect AAA but cannot rule out rupture reliably.
- CT is diagnostic in 95% of patients with acute abdominal pain.

ABC approach to evaluation + workup of abdominal pain (ED/AMU):

A — Assess severity & immediate threats

Goal: identify "sick vs not sick" + time-critical diagnoses.

- **Vitals + NEWS2:** HR, BP, RR, SpO$_2$, temp, mental state, urine output.
- **Red flags (treat as emergency):**
  - **Shock/syncope**, persistent tachycardia, **hypotension**
  - **Peritonism** (rigid/guarding/rebound)
  - **GI bleed** (melaena/PR bleeding/haematemesis)
  - **Pregnancy** / vaginal bleeding
  - **Pain out of proportion** (mesenteric ischaemia)
  - **AAA risk** (older, smoker, back pain, collapse)
- **Immediate actions** (while assessing): 2 wide-bore IV, **bloods + VBG/ABG lactate**, analgesia, antiemetic, fluids, **sepsis 6** if septic, early senior/surgical/OBGYN input if indicated.

B — Bedside assessment

Goal: get high-yield clues quickly.

- **Focused history (SOCRATES + key associates):**
  - Onset (sudden vs gradual), site/radiation (back/shoulder/groin), character (colicky vs constant), severity, progression
  - **Vomiting**, bowel habit/obstruction symptoms, PR bleeding/melaena
  - **Urinary** symptoms/loin pain, **fever**, **jaundice**
  - **Gynae:** LMP, contraception, vaginal bleeding/discharge, pregnancy risk

- PMH: AF/PVD (ischaemia), gallstones/alcohol (pancreatitis), peptic ulcer/NSAIDs, previous surgery/hernia (obstruction)
- **Exam (don't skip the basics):**
    - General: hydration, jaundice, pallor, distress
    - Abdomen: distension, scars, hernias → tenderness, guarding, masses, pulsatile mass
    - **PR** if bleeding/obstruction suspected
    - **Testes** in males with lower abdominal pain
    - Chest exam if upper abdominal pain (pneumonia/PE can mimic)

C — Core investigations (workup)

Goal: rule in/out common & dangerous causes; guide imaging.

1) Must-do early for many patients

- **ECG** (especially epigastric/upper abdo pain, older, diabetic)
- **Urine dip** (blood/nitrite/ketones)
- **β-hCG in all women of childbearing potential** (don't rely on history alone)

2) Blood tests (typical acute panel)

- **FBC, U&E/Cr, CRP**
- **LFTs** (biliary/hepatic)
- **Lipase/amylase** (pancreatitis)
- **VBG/ABG lactate** (shock/ischaemia/sepsis)
- **Clotting, group & save ± crossmatch** if bleeding/AAA/operative risk
- **Glucose** ± ketones if diabetic/unwell

3) Imaging (choose based on pattern)
- CT Abdomen/Pelvis (often CT with contrast) if:
  - severe/undifferentiated pain, **peritonism**, suspected **obstruction, appendicitis** unclear, **perforation, ischaemia**, complicated diverticulitis
- **RUQ ultrasound:** gallstones/cholecystitis/cholangitis, biliary dilatation
- **CT KUB (non-contrast):** renal colic
- **CXR:** free air (perforation), pneumonia
- **CT angiography:** suspected **AAA** or **mesenteric ischaemia**

4) Targeted extras (as indicated)
- **Blood cultures** if fever/sepsis
- **Stool tests** if infectious diarrhoea/IBD flare
- **Pelvic USS** if gynae pathology suspected
- **Troponin** if cardiac cause possible

Quick "pattern → likely test"
- **RUQ pain + fever/jaundice** → LFTs, cultures, **RUQ USS** (± MRCP/ERCP pathway)
- **Epigastric to back** → lipase, LFTs, calcium/TG if pancreatitis, CT if severe/uncertain
- **Colicky distension + vomiting + no stool/flatus** → CT A/P (obstruction)

  Loin → groin + haematuria → CT KUB
- **Older + AF + pain out of proportion + ↑lactate** → **CT angiography** (mesenteric ischaemia)
- **Reproductive-age + pain ± bleeding** → β-hCG first, then pelvic USS/OBGYN

Mnemonic: Abdominal Pain causes- **ABDOMINAL**

- **A** appendicitis
- **B** biliary tract disease
- **D** diverticulitis
- **O** ovarian disease
- **M** malignancy 🚩
- **I** intestinal obstruction 🚩
- **N** nephritic syndrome
- **A** acute pancreatitis 🚩
- **L** liquor (ethanol)

Mnemonic: Abdominal distension causes: 6 F

1. **Fat:** e.g. obesity
2. **Fluid:** e.g. ascites or cyst (ovarian or pseudo-pancreatic cyst)
3. **Flatus:** e.g. abdominal distension
4. **Feces:** e.g. intestinal obstruction
5. **Fetus:** e.g. pregnancy
6. **Fatal tumour** e.g. malignancy

📖 Mnemonic for red flags for acute abdominal pain : SHOCK

S – Sepsis / Severe infection
- Peritonitis, perforated viscus, appendicitis with abscess, cholangitis

H – Haemorrhage
- Ruptured AAA
- Ruptured ectopic pregnancy
- GI bleed (massive haematemesis, melaena)

O – Obstruction
- Bowel obstruction with vomiting, distension, no flatus
- Strangulated hernia

C – Critical ischaemia
- Mesenteric ischaemia ("pain out of proportion")
- Ischaemic colitis

K – Killers (malignancy / masses)
- Colorectal cancer with ± obstruction
- Ovarian / pelvic mass with torsion

Back pain

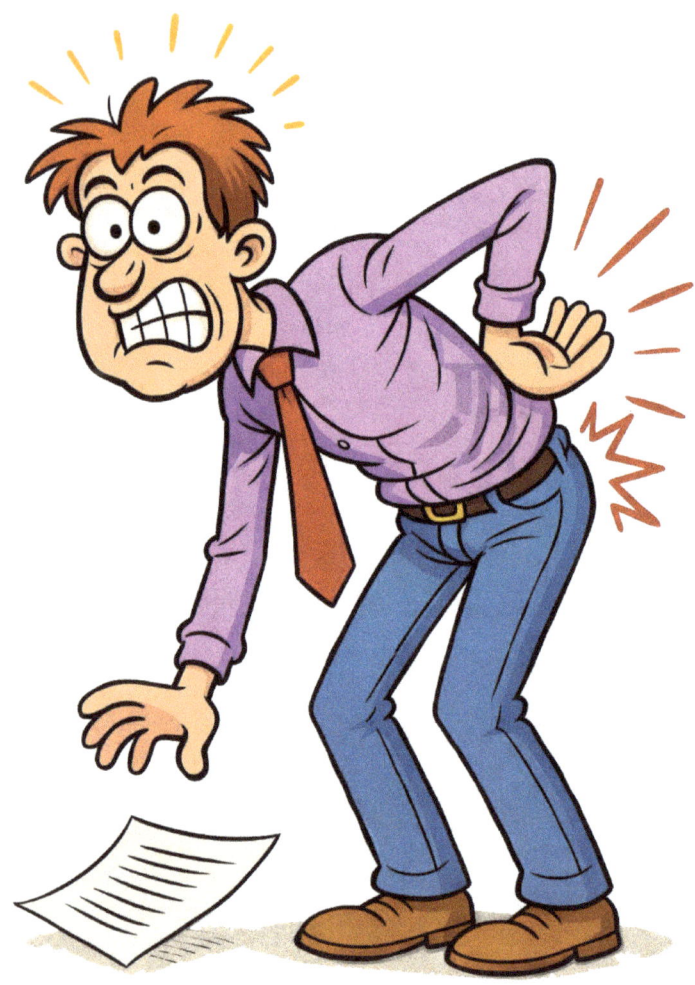

🚩 Red Flags: Back pain

> ⚠ Age 55 with new-onset back pain.
> ⚠ History of cancer
> ⚠ Unexplained weight loss
> ⚠ Persistent /progressive pain (night pain, not relieved by rest)
> ⚠ Fever, night sweats, rigors
> ⚠ Immunosuppressants (HIV, Steroids, transplant, IV drug use)
> ⚠ History of trauma (esp. elderly/osteoporotic)
> ⚠ Neurological symptoms (weakness, numbness, saddle anesthesia)
> ⚠ New bladder/bowel dysfunction (urinary/faecal incontinence)
> ⚠ Spinal deformity (kyphosis, scoliosis, step deformity)
> ⚠ Corticosteroid use/osteoporosis
> ⚠ Unremitting pain at rest/night pain

∏ Age < 20 or >55 with new-onset back pain:
- **Implications/Diagnoses:** Serious pathology, not simple mechanical pain-Malignancy, Infection.
- **Investigations:** MRI spine, X-ray, CT, bone scan, myeloma screen, blood cultures, ESR, CRP.

∏ History of cancer:
- **Implications/Diagnoses:** Metastatic disease to spine.
- **Investigations:** MRI Spine, CT spine, PET-CT, biopsy.

∏ Unexplained weight loss:
- **Implications/Diagnoses:** Malignancy or infection.
- **Investigations:** MRI spine, myeloma screen (serum electrophoresis, skeletal survey), QuantiFERON TB culture, biopsy.

∏ Persistent/progressive pain (esp., night pain, not relieved by rest) :
- **Implications/Diagnoses:** Non-mechanical cause- Malignancy, Infection, inflammatory spondyloarthropathy.
- **Investigations:** MRI spine, CT, tumour markers, ESR/CRP, blood cultures, Pelvic X-ray, MRI sacroiliac joints, HLA-B27, CRP.

∏ Fever, night sweats, rigors:
- **Implications/Diagnoses:** Infection- Osteomyelitis/discitis, Epidural abscess.
- **Investigations:** MRI spine with contrast, ESR/CRP, blood cultures.
- Urgent neurosurgical review.

∏ Immunosuppression (HIV, transplant, IV drug use, diabetes):
- **Implications/Diagnoses:** High risk spinal infection- Discitis, Osteomyelitis.
- **Investigations:**MRI spine, ESR/CRP, blood cultures, biopsy for microbiology.

∏ History of trauma (esp. elderly/osteoporotic) :
- **Implications/Diagnoses:** vertebral compression fracture.
- **Investigations:** X-ray spine, CT spine, DEXA scan (for osteoporosis).

⨿ Neurological symptoms (weakness, numbness, bilateral sciatica, saddle anesthesia):

- **Implications/Diagnoses:** Cord or cauda equina involvement- Cauda equina syndrome, Spinal cord compression.
- **Investigations:** MRI whole spine, MRI lumbar spine, bladder scan (retention), post-void residuals.
- Urgent neurosurgery input.

⨿ New bladder/bowel dysfunction (urinary retention, Incontinence, faecal incontinence):

- **Implications/Diagnoses:** Cauda Equina Syndrome.
- **Investigations:** MRI lumbar spine, bladder scan.
- Urgent neurosurgical referral.

⨿ Spinal deformity (kyphosis, scoliosis, step deformity):

- **Implications/Diagnoses:** structural cause-Fracture, Spondylolisthesis, Malignancy/infection.
- **Investigations:** X-ray, CT spine, MRI spine, biopsy.

⨿ Corticosteroid use/osteoporosis:

- **Implications/Diagnoses:** Vertebral fracture.
- **Investigations:** X-ray, MRI spine, DEXA screen.

⨿ Unremitting pain at rest/night pain:

- **Implications/Diagnoses:** Malignancy, infection, or inflammatory arthritis.
- **Investigations:** MRI spine, MRI sacroiliac joints, bone scan, ESR/CRP, blood cultures, HLA-B27.

🔑 Key Points:

1. Red flags- urgent MRI spine is often first-line.
2.
3. Blood tests (FBC, ESR, CRP) and plain X-rays help, but MRI is the gold standard for ruling out malignancy, infection and cord compression.
4. AAA should be considered in any elderly patient with low back pain.
5. Most spinal disorders are mechanical. Only a few involve infection, inflammation, or cancer (non-mechanical).
6. Serious spinal disorders are – Infections (e.g. discitis, epidural abscess, osteomyelitis), Primary tumors-(spinal cord or vertebrae), Metastatic vertebral tumors (most often from breasts, Lungs or prostate).
7. Mechanical spine disorders can be serious if they compress the spinal nerve roots or particularly the spinal cord.
8. Spinal cord compression can happen due to disorders such as tumors, epidural abscess or hematoma.

ABC approach to evaluation + workup of back pain (ED/AMU):

A — Assess severity & "can't-miss" emergencies
Immediate red flags (act now):

- **Cauda equina:** new urinary retention/overflow, faecal incontinence, saddle anaesthesia, bilateral sciatica, severe/progressive weakness
- **Spinal cord compression:** progressive neuro deficit, gait disturbance
- **Spinal infection** (discitis/osteomyelitis/epidural abscess): **fever**, IVDU, immunosuppression, recent bacteraemia/procedure, severe constant night pain

- **Fracture:** major trauma, minor trauma in **osteoporosis**, prolonged steroids
- **Malignancy:** history of cancer, **weight loss**, night pain, age >50 with new severe pain
- **AAA / vascular catastrophe:** older, smoker, collapse, hypotension, severe back/abdo pain
- **Renal/visceral mimic:** flank pain, haematuria, urinary symptoms, RUQ/epigastric pain, chest pain

Immediate actions if unwell/neurology present
- Vitals/NEWS2, analgesia early, IV access if septic/shocked
- Full **neurology** + bladder scan if retention suspected
- Escalate urgently (spinal/ortho/neurosurgery; med reg; vascular; O&G if pregnant)

B — Bedside assessment

1) Focused history
- Onset (sudden after strain vs spontaneous), location, radiation (sciatica), severity, progression
- **Neuro symptoms:** weakness, numbness, saddle symptoms, gait, falls
- **Bladder/bowel/sexual** dysfunction
- Systemic: fever, weight loss, night sweats
- Risk: cancer, IVDU, immunosuppression, diabetes, TB risk, anticoagulants
- Trauma/osteoporosis/steroid use
- Pregnancy, abdominal symptoms, urinary symptoms

2) Examination

- Observe gait, posture; inspect spine
- Palpate midline tenderness
- **Neuro exam (must document):**
  - Power (hip flexion, knee extension, ankle dorsiflex/plantarflex, big toe ext)
  - Reflexes (knee, ankle), sensation incl. **saddle area**
  - Straight leg raise/slump (radiculopathy)
- **Perianal sensation + anal tone** if cauda equina suspected
- Abdominal exam ± **AAA palpation** (don't rely on this to exclude)
- Consider hip exam if pain may be referred

C — Core investigations (workup)

Most uncomplicated mechanical back pain: usually no tests initially.

Do these when red flags, systemic features, significant neuro deficit, trauma, or atypical pain:

1) Bedside

- **Urine dip** (haematuria/infection)
- **Pregnancy test** if relevant
- **Bladder scan** if urinary symptoms/possible retention

2) Bloods

- If infection/malignancy/inflammatory concern: **FBC, CRP/ESR, U&E**
- **Blood cultures** if febrile/septic
- Consider **PSA** (men with malignancy features), **calcium** if malignancy suspected (context-dependent)

3) **Imaging (choose the right one)**
- **MRI whole spine (urgent, same day) if:**
  - suspected **cauda equina**
  - suspected **cord compression**
  - suspected **spinal epidural abscess/discitis**
  - severe/progressive neuro deficit
  - suspected malignancy with neuro signs
- **CT spine if:**
  - suspected **fracture** (esp. trauma) or MRI unavailable for bony detail
- **Plain X-ray:** limited value; consider mainly for trauma/osteoporosis suspicion (not for routine non-specific pain)
- **CT angiography** if **AAA** suspected
- **CT KUB** if renal colic suspected (flank pain + haematuria)

Practical "pattern → next step"
- **Back pain + urinary retention/saddle anaesthesia →** bladder scan + urgent MRI + emergency referral
- **Back pain + fever/IVDU/immunosuppressed →** bloods + cultures + urgent MRI
- **New back pain + cancer history/weight loss/night pain →** urgent MRI (or CT per local pathway)
- **Trauma/osteoporosis/steroids + midline tenderness →** CT (± X-ray) for fracture
- **Older smoker + sudden severe back pain/collapse →** resus + CT angiography (AAA)

Mnemonic causes of back pain : Back Pain

B – Bone pathology 🚩
- Metastatic cancer
- Multiple myeloma
- Fractures (osteoporotic, traumatic, pathological)

A – Abdominal aortic aneurysm (AAA) 🚩
- Sudden tearing back pain, shock

C – Cauda equina syndrome 🚩
- Saddle anaesthesia, incontinence, leg weakness

K – Kidney causes
- Pyelonephritis
- Renal stones (renal colic)

P – Prolapsed disc / spinal stenosis (common)
- Radiculopathy, sciatica

A – Ankylosing spondylitis / inflammatory arthritis
- Young patient, morning stiffness, improves with activity

I – Infection 🚩
- Spinal epidural abscess
- Discitis, vertebral osteomyelitis
- TB spine (Pott's disease)

N – Neurological disorders / Non-mechanical causes
- Demyelination
- Syringomyelia

Mnemonic for red flag of back pain: "TUNIS"

- **T** – Trauma (fracture)
- **U** – Unexplained weight loss / cancer history (malignancy, myeloma, mets)
- **N** – Neurology (cauda equina, progressive deficit, saddle anaesthesia, incontinence)
- **I** – Infection (discitis, abscess, TB spine)
- **S** – Serious vascular (AAA, retroperitoneal bleed)

Chest Pain

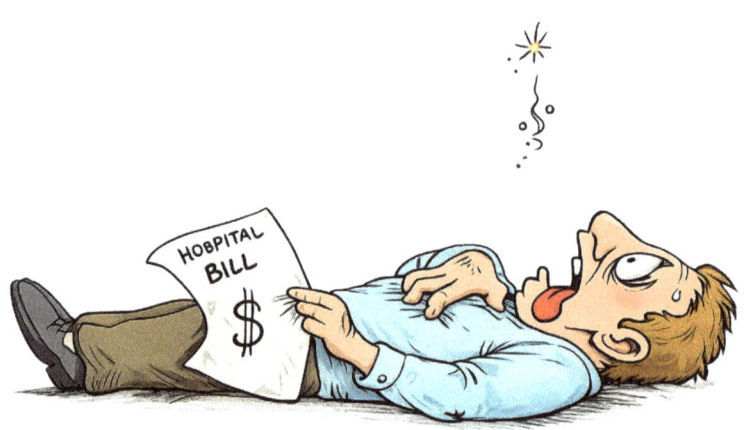

▶ Red Flags: Chest Pain

- ⚠ **Confusion**
- ⚠ **Absent breath sounds**
- ⚠ **New ECG changes**
- ⚠ **Central, crushing, or pressure-like chest pain ± radiation**
- ⚠ **Sudden, severe "tearing/ripping" chest or back pain**
- ⚠ **Associated syncope, dizziness, or severe hypotension**
- ⚠ **Associated dyspnoea, haemoptysis, pleuritic pain**
- ⚠ **Pain with fever, rigors, or productive cough**
- ⚠ **Severe, sharp, pleuritic pain with acute dyspnea**
- ⚠ **Positional chest pain (worse lying flat, better sitting forward)**
- ⚠ **Unequal arm blood pressures or new neurological deficit**
- ⚠ **Known risk factors (diabetes, hypertension, smoking, family history of CAD) with new onset chest pain**
- ⚠ **Chest pain in a patient with cancer, immunosuppression, HIV or IV drug use**
- ⚠ **Severe chest pain with shock, muffled heart sounds, distended neck veins (Beck's triad)**

∏ **Confusion/Delerium:**
- ❖ **Implications/Diagnoses:** Pneumonia, Cholecystitis, other infections
- ❖ **Investigations:** Sepsis screen, CXR, blood cultures. LFT, USS abdomen.

∏ Absent breath sounds on auscultation:
* **Implications/Diagnoses:** Pneumothorax, Pleural effusion.
* **Investigations:** CXR, CT chest.

∏ New ECG changes:
* **Implications/Diagnoses:** MI, PE
* **Investigations:** ECG- Look for S1Q3T3 pattern, new sinus tachycardia, T wave inversions, new onset LBBB, ST elevation.
* Check troponin (can be positive in MI & PE) / D-dimer. Urgent CT Pulmonary angiogram if no cause is found. Cardiology referral, if possible, ACS.

∏ Central, crushing, or pressure-like chest pain ± radiation (jaw, arm, back):
* **Implications/Diagnoses:** Acute coronary syndrome (ACS), STEMI, NSTEMI, unstable angina.
* **Investigations:** ECG (ST/T changes, new LBBB), serial troponins, CXR, angiogram.

∏ Sudden, severe "tearing/ripping" chest pain or back pain :
* **Implications/Diagnoses:** Aortic pathology- Aortic dissection, ruptured thoracic aneurysm.
* **Investigations:** CT aortogram, ECG (to rule out MI), CXR (Widened mediastinum), echocardiogram.

∏ Associated syncope, dizziness, or severe hypotension :
* **Implications/Diagnoses:** Cardiovascular Collapse-Massive PE, aortic dissection, MI with arrhythmia, cardiac tamponade.
* **Investigations:** ECG, troponin, echocardiogram, CTPA (if PE suspected), ABG, lactate.

∏ Associated dyspnoea, haemoptysis, pleuritic pain:

- **Implications/Diagnoses:** PE, Pneumonia, Pneumothorax.
- **Investigations:** Well's score, D-dimer, CTPA, V/Q scan (if CTPA contraindicated), ECG (S1Q3T3 pattern, RBBB, T wave inversions), CXR, USS leg doppler, CRP/WBC.

∏ Pain with fever, rigors, or productive cough:

- **Implications/Diagnoses:** Pneumonia, empyema, pericarditis(if positional/pleuritic).
- **Investigations:** FBC(neutrophilia), CRP, blood cultures, sputum cultures, CXR, ECG (pericarditis), echocardiogram.

∏ Severe, sharp, pleuritic pain with acute dyspnoea:

- **Implications/Diagnoses:** Pneumothorax, PE, pleural effusion.
- **Investigations:** CXR, USS(pleural fluid), ABG, CTPA (if PE suspected).

∏ Positional chest pain (worse lying flat, better sitting forward):

- **Implications/Diagnoses:** Pericardial Inflammation-Pericarditis.
- **Investigations:** ECG (widespread ST elevation, PR depression), echocardiogram (effusion), troponin (myopericarditis), CRP/ESR.

∏ Unequal arm blood pressures or new neurological deficit:

- **Implications/Diagnoses:** Aortic dissection.
- **Investigations:** CT aortogram, echocardiogram, CXR, Doppler/angiography of affected vessels.

∏ Known risk factors (diabetes, hypertension, smoking, family history of CAD) with new chest pain :

- **Implications/Diagnoses:** ACS, Stable angina.
- **Investigations:** ECG, troponin, ETT, stress echo , CT coronary angiogram.

∏ Chest pain in a patient with cancer, immunosuppression, or IV drug use:

- ❖ **Implications/Diagnoses:** Infection, malignancy- Lung cancer, septic pulmonary emboli, infective endocarditis with septic emboli, mediastinitis.
- ❖ **Investigations:** CXR, CT chest, blood cultures, echocardiogram (endocarditis), bronchoscopy/biopsy(if cancer suspected).

∏ Severe chest pain with shock, muffled heart sounds, distended neck veins (Beck's triad):

- ❖ **Implications/Diagnoses:** Cardiac tamponade/Pericardial effusion.
- ❖ **Investigations:** echocardiogram, ECG (low voltage, QRS, electrical alternans), CXR (globular heart).
- ❖ Urgent pericardiocentesis.

🔑 Key points:

- Immediate tests in all chest pain: ECG+troponin+CXR+bloods.
- Definitive imaging depends on suspected cause: CT aortogram(dissection), CTPA(PE), Echo(tamponade/pericarditis), angiogram(ACS).
- Rule out immediately life-threatening causes: ACS, Thoracic aortic dissection, Tension Pneumothorax, Esophageal rupture, Pulmonary embolism.
- Coronary ischaemia and PE may not have a "classical" presentation.

ABC approach to evaluation + workup of chest pain (ED/AMU)

A — Assess immediately (sick vs not sick)

Do first (within minutes):

- **Vitals/NEWS2:** HR, BP (both arms if possible), RR, SpO_2, temp, conscious level
- **Immediate ECG** (aim **within 10 minutes**) + put on monitor
- Quick look for **instability**: hypotension, hypoxia, arrhythmia, altered mental state, ongoing severe pain, diaphoresis

Time-critical "can't miss" causes

- **ACS / MI**
- **Pulmonary embolism**
- **Aortic dissection**
- **Tension pneumothorax**
- **Cardiac tamponade**
- **Oesophageal rupture** (severe pain after vomiting, mediastinal emphysema/sepsis)

If unstable: resus ABC, senior help early, treat suspected diagnosis in parallel with tests.

B — Bedside assessment (focused history + exam)

1) Focused history (high yield)

- **Pain:** onset (sudden vs gradual), character (tight/pressure/pleuritic/tearing), location/radiation (arm/jaw/back), duration, triggers (exertion), relief (GTN), severity

- **Associated symptoms:** breathlessness, syncope, palpitations, nausea/vomiting, sweating, haemoptysis, fever, cough
- **Risk factors**
  - ACS: age, diabetes, smoking, HTN, HLD, family history
  - PE: recent immobilisation/surgery, cancer, OCP/HRT, prior VTE
  - Dissection: HTN, connective tissue disease, known aneurysm
- **Mimics:** reflux, anxiety/panic, musculoskeletal strain, shingles prodrome

2) Exam

- CVS: heart sounds (murmur), JVP, peripheral perfusion
- Resp: asymmetric breath sounds, creps, wheeze
- Legs: DVT signs
- Chest wall: reproducible tenderness (doesn't fully exclude ACS)
- Skin: rash (zoster)

C — Core investigations (workup)

1) Must-do for almost everyone

- **ECG:** repeat if ongoing pain or initial non-diagnostic
- **Bloods: high-sensitivity troponin** (0/1h or 0/2–3h pathway per local), **FBC, U&E, CRP**, glucose
- **Chest X-ray** (pneumothorax, pneumonia, widened mediastinum, effusion)
- **VBG/ABG** if hypoxic, shocked, or very breathless (lactate helpful)

2) Targeted tests by suspicion

- **PE:** Wells (or Geneva) → **D-dimer** if low/intermediate risk; **CTPA** if high risk or D-dimer positive; consider leg ultrasound if needed
- **Aortic dissection:** urgent **CT aortogram/CTA** if suspected (tearing pain, neuro deficit, pulse/BP differential, mediastinal widening)
- **Pericarditis:** ECG changes + raised inflammatory markers; consider echo
- **Heart failure/strain:** BNP (if uncertain), echo
- **Pneumothorax:** CXR or bedside ultrasound if unstable
- **Oesophageal rupture:** CT chest with contrast (and urgent senior/surgical input)

3) "Second-line" cardiac imaging (selected patients)

- **CT coronary angiography** (CTCA): low–intermediate risk chest pain where ACS unclear (per local pathway)
- **Echocardiography:** suspected tamponade, RV strain (massive PE), new murmur/mechanical complication, LV dysfunction

Quick pattern → likely pathway

- **Pressure/tightness + exertional + risk factors** → ACS workup (serial ECG + troponin ± cardiology)
- **Pleuritic pain + SOB ± haemoptysis + VTE risk** → PE pathway (Wells/D-dimer/CTPA)
- **Sudden tearing chest/back pain ± neuro signs/BP differential** → Dissection (CTA)

- **Unilateral pleuritic pain + reduced breath sounds** → Pneumothorax (CXR/US)
- **Sharp pain better sitting forward + pericardial rub** → Pericarditis (ECG/CRP ± echo)

📋 Mnemonic for causes of Life-threatening chest pain: **DEATH**

- **D** Dissection(aortic)
- **E** Embolism(pulmonary)
- **A** Acute coronary syndrome
- **T** Tamponade
- **H** Hole in Gut (esophageal perforation)

📋 Mnemonic for Causes of Chest Pain: **"CHEST PAINS"**

👉 **Covers common & serious causes together**

C – Coronary syndromes 🚩
- ACS (STEMI, NSTEMI, unstable angina)

H – Heart failure / pericardial disease
- Pericarditis, pericardial effusion 🚩

E – Embolism 🚩
- Pulmonary embolism

S – Spasm / Oesophageal
- GORD, oesophageal spasm, reflux oesophagitis

T – Trauma / MSK
- Costochondritis, rib fracture, muscle strain

P – Pneumothorax / Pleural disease 🚩
- Tension pneumothorax, pleurisy

A – Aortic catastrophe 🚩

- Aortic dissection, ruptured aneurysm

I – Infection (pulmonary)

- Pneumonia, TB

N – Non-cardiac anxiety / panic attacks

- Functional chest pain

S – Stomach / upper GI

- Peptic ulcer, gastritis, biliary colic, pancreatitis 🚩

📖 Mnemonic for Red Flags in Chest Pain: "PAINS RED" ❌

👉 The must-not-miss killers

P – PE / Pneumothorax (tension)

A – ACS / Angina (unstable) / MI

I – Infection severe (sepsis from pneumonia, mediastinitis)

N – Non-traumatic dissection / rupture (Aortic dissection, ruptured aneurysm)

S – Shock states (pericardial tamponade, massive haemothorax)

R – Radiating pain to arm/jaw/back (classic ACS/dissection)

E – Elderly or at-risk (diabetes, HTN, cancer) with sudden pain

D – Dangerous deterioration (hypotension, hypoxia, syncope)

Constipation

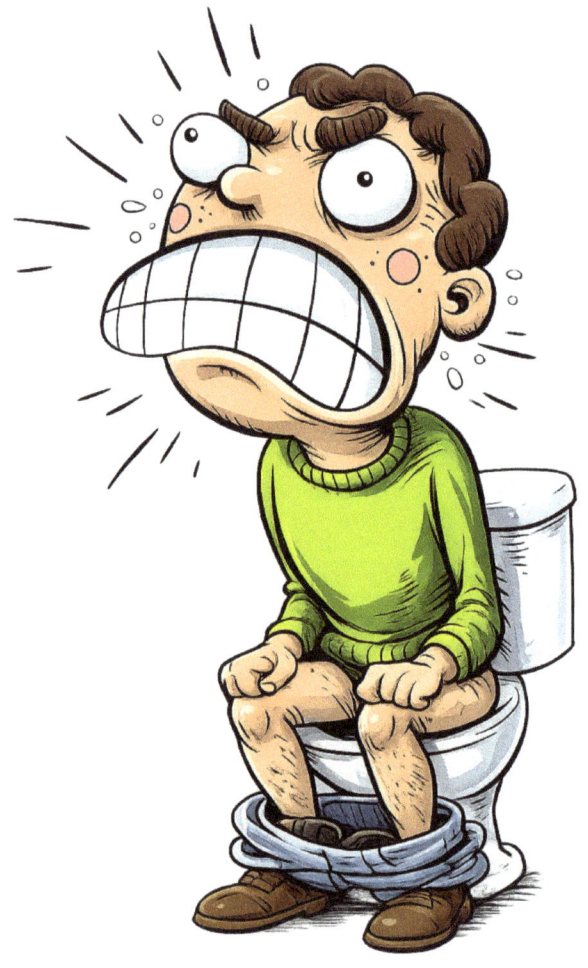

Red Flags: Constipation

- ⚠ **Unintentional weight loss**
- ⚠ **Iron-deficiency anaemia/rectal bleeding**
- ⚠ **New-onset constipation in patients > 50 years**
- ⚠ **Family history of colorectal cancer/polyposis syndromes**
- ⚠ **Change in bowel habits (constipation alternating with diarrhea)**
- ⚠ **Abdominal pain/distension, vomiting, bloating or palpable mass**
- ⚠ **Persistent constipation despite laxatives**
- ⚠ **Neurological symptoms (saddle anesthesia, urinary retention)**
- ⚠ **Constitutional symptoms (fever, night sweats, anorexia)**
- ⚠ **Long term opioid use/systemic illness**
- ⚠ **Sudden cognitive impairment in elderly**

∏ Unintentional weight loss:
- ❖ **Implications/Diagnoses:** Colorectal cancer, Pancreatic cancer, Endocrine/metabolic.
- ❖ **Investigations:** Colonoscopy with biopsy, CT abdomen/pelvis, CT colonography, CEA tumour marker, MRI pancreas/ERCP, TSH, calcium, glucose, cortisol.

∏ Iron-deficiency anaemia/rectal bleeding:
- **Implications/Diagnoses:** Colorectal cancer, IBD, Hemorrhoids, fissures.
- **Investigations:** Colonoscopy with biopsy, FIT/FOBT, CT colonography, faecal calprotectin, CRP, sigmoidoscopy.

∏ New-onset constipation in patients > 50 years:
- **Implications/Diagnoses:** Colorectal cancer/strictures, Diverticular disease.
- **Investigations:** Colonoscopy ± biopsy, CT colonography, CT abdomen/pelvis.

∏ Family history of colorectal cancer/polyposis syndromes:
- **Implications/Diagnoses:** Hereditary /Sporadic colorectal cancer.
- **Investigations:** Colonoscopy, biopsy, CT staging, surveillance.

∏ Change in bowel habit (constipation, alternating with diarrhoea):
- **Implications/Diagnoses:** Colorectal cancer, IBD, diverticular strictures.
- **Investigations:** Colonoscopy with biopsy, CT colonography, faecal calprotectin, flexible sigmoidoscopy.

∏ Abdominal pain/distension, vomiting, bloating, or palpable mass:
- **Implications/Diagnoses:** Colorectal cancer, Volvulus, Ovarian mass, Faecal impaction, bowel obstruction, diverticulitis.
- **Investigations:** Colonoscopy, biopsy, CT abdomen/pelvis, AXR, sigmoidoscopy, USS pelvis/abdomen, CA-125, MRI pelvis, digital rectal exam.

∏ Persistent constipation despite laxatives:

- **Implications/Diagnoses:** Colorectal cancer, Neurological conditions (Parkinson's, MS), Endocrine/metabolic.
- **Investigations:** TSH, calcium, glucose, cortisol, Colonoscopy, CT colonography, MRI bran/spine.

∏ Neurological symptoms (saddle anaesthesia, weakness, urinary retention) :

- **Implications/Diagnoses:** Cauda equina syndrome, spinal cord compression.
- **Investigations:** MRI whole spine, MRI lumbar spine, bladder scan (post-void residuals), CT if MRI contraindicated.
- Neurosurgical review.

∏ Constitutional symptoms (fever, night sweats, anorexia):

- **Implications/Diagnoses:** IBD, Malignancy, Intra-abdominal abscess/TB.
- **Investigations:** Colonoscopy with biopsy, CT abdomen/pelvis, CRP, faecal calprotectin, TB cultures, biopsy.

∏ Long-term opioid use/systemic illness:

- **Implications/Diagnoses:** Opioid-induced constipation, Endocrine/metabolic, Neurological.
- **Investigations:** AXR, CT abdomen, TSH, cortisol, calcium, glucose, MRI spine/brain if focal deficits.

∏ Sudden cognitive impairment in elderly:

- **Implications/Diagnoses:** faecal impaction, electrolyte imbalance.
- **Investigations:** UEC, digital rectum examination, CT brain if no explanation.

🔑 Key points:

- Always investigate red flags constipation with colonoscopy ± biopsy.
- CT colonography is alternative if colonoscopy is not possible.
- MRI spine is urgent in any neurological red flag (cauda equina).
- Acute constipation suggests an organic cause most commonly- bowel obstruction, adynamic ileus, drugs.
- Be wary of bowel obstruction when constipation is acute and severe particularly when associated with vomiting/abdominal distension.
- Drugs causes are common (e.g. chronic laxative abuse, use of anticholinergic or opioid drugs).

ABC approach to constipation (evaluation + workup):

A — Assessment and immediate threats (rule out "can't miss")

Triage severity

- Vitals/NEWS2, hydration, pain score, vomiting, ability to tolerate PO.

Immediate threats / red flags (urgent same-day workup)

- **Suspected bowel obstruction: absolute constipation** (no stool *and* no flatus), severe colicky pain, **progressive distension**, persistent vomiting
- **Peritonism / perforation:** guarding, rebound, rigid abdomen, sepsis
- **Malignancy/serious pathology: new constipation >50**, rapid change in bowel habit, **weight loss, PR bleeding, iron-deficiency anaemia**

- **Severe faecal impaction:** overflow diarrhoea, severe rectal pain, urinary retention, confusion (frail)
- **Neurology red flags:** new leg weakness, saddle anaesthesia, new bladder/bowel dysfunction
- **High-risk patient:** immunosuppressed, significant comorbidity, pregnancy (consider causes/med safety)

Immediate actions if any red flag

- IV access ± fluids; **NBM** if obstruction suspected
- **Abdominal exam + PR exam**
- **Bloods:** FBC, U&E, CRP, LFT, **calcium** ± glucose/TSH
- **Imaging: CT abdomen/pelvis** if obstruction/perforation/mass suspected (AXR only if CT not available)
- Early senior/surgical review if obstruction or peritonism

B — Bedside assessment (focused history and exam)

Focused history

- **Time course:** acute vs chronic; baseline bowel habit
- **Symptoms:** stool frequency, Bristol type, straining, incomplete emptying, sensation of blockage, manual manoeuvres
- **Associated:** abdominal pain/bloating, nausea/vomiting, rectal pain, bleeding, weight loss, fever
- **Diet/fluids/mobility:** low intake, immobility, poor toileting access, suppressed urge
- **Medication review (very common):**
  - **Opioids**, anticholinergics (TCAs/oxybutynin), antipsychotics
  - **Iron**, calcium, **verapamil**, ondansetron, antihistamines, diuretics (dehydration)

- **Secondary causes screen:**
  - **Endocrine/metabolic:** hypothyroid, **hypercalcaemia**, diabetes
  - **Neuro:** Parkinson's, MS, stroke, spinal disease
  - **Structural/anorectal:** fissure, haemorrhoids, prolapse, rectocele; FHx bowel cancer
- **Red flag check:** new onset >50, anaemia, weight loss, PR bleed, nocturnal symptoms, TB/systemic features if relevant

Focused exam

- **General:** hydration, cachexia, confusion, mobility
- **Abdominal:** distension, masses, tenderness, bowel sounds, hernias
- **PR exam (key):**
  - **Impaction**, rectal mass, blood, fissure/haemorrhoids
  - Anal tone + neuro screen if indicated

C- Core investigations (workup)

If likely functional constipation and no red flags

Often **no tests initially**. If persistent/recurrent, older, frail, or secondary cause suspected:

- **FBC** (anaemia), **U&E** (dehydration/AKI), **calcium**
- **TSH** (chronic/refractory) ± glucose/HbA1c if diabetes suspected

If acute severe symptoms or red flags

- **FBC**, **U&E**, **CRP**, LFT, **calcium** ± lactate/VBG if systemically unwell
- **CT abdomen/pelvis** if obstruction/perforation/mass suspected

If chronic constipation with alarm features
- Follow local pathway: **FIT** (where appropriate) and/or **2-week-wait colorectal referral**
- **Colonoscopy** or **CT colonography** depending on suitability

If refractory constipation / suspected outlet obstruction (secondary care)
- **Transit studies** (marker study), **anorectal manometry, balloon expulsion test**
- **Defecography** if pelvic floor dysfunction suspected

Management "while you work it up" (brief, practical)
- **Treat impaction first:** PR confirms → **rectal therapy** (glycerin/bisacodyl suppository or phosphate enema if safe) ± **high-dose macrogol** regimen
- **Osmotic first-line: macrogol (PEG)**; add **stimulant** (senna/bisacodyl) if needed
- **Avoid bulking agents** if **suspected obstruction**, severe slow-transit with bloating, or poor fluid intake
- **Opioid constipation:** stimulant + PEG; consider **peripherally acting µ-opioid antagonist** per local policy if refractory
- Lifestyle: fluids, fibre (if appropriate), mobilise, toileting routine after meals, footstool (defaecation posture)

📖 Mnemonic for Causes of Constipation: "STOOL BLOCK"

👉 Covers common & serious causes

S – Structural
- Colorectal cancer 🚩
- Strictures (IBD, radiation, diverticular disease)

T – Toxins / Drugs
- Opiates 🚩
- Anticholinergics (TCAs, antihistamines)
- Iron supplements, CCBs

O – Obstruction outside colon
- Pelvic / ovarian mass 🚩
- Pregnancy

O – Old age
- Reduced mobility, dehydration, diet changes

L – Lifestyle factors
- Low fibre diet, inactivity

B – Brain & spinal cord disease 🚩
- Parkinson's, MS, spinal cord injury

L – Low thyroid (hypothyroidism)
- Metabolic: hypercalcaemia, diabetes

O – Outlet dysfunction
- Anal fissure, haemorrhoids, rectal prolapse

C – Congenital / Childhood
- Hirschsprung's disease 🚩
- Cystic fibrosis

K – Kidney disease
- **CKD with electrolyte imbalance**

📋 Mnemonic for Red Flags in Constipation: "CRAMPS"

C – Change in bowel habit (esp. new-onset in >50 yrs)

R – Rectal bleeding / anaemia

A – Abdominal mass or weight loss

M – Medication resistant / persistent symptoms

P – Pain at night / severe abdominal pain

S – Symptoms of obstruction (vomiting, distension, no flatus)

✅ How to remember
- **"STOOL BLOCK"** → think of a blocked stool = causes
- **"CRAMPS"** → think of painful cramps = red flags

Cough

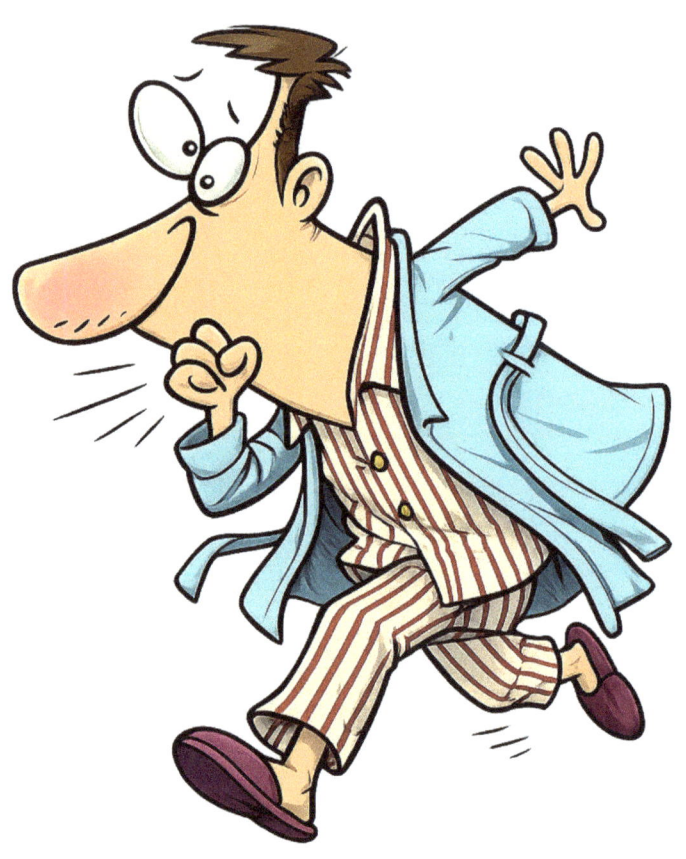

▶ Red Flags: Cough

- ⚠ Haemoptysis
- ⚠ Unintentional weight loss, anorexia, night sweats
- ⚠ Persistent cough > 8 weeks, not improving
- ⚠ Smoking history (>40 yrs) with new/changing cough
- ⚠ Dyspnoea, pleuritic chest pain, haemoptysis (classic PE triad)
- ⚠ Fever, rigors, productive purulent sputum, pleuritic pain
- ⚠ Clubbing or chronic purulent sputum production
- ⚠ Stridor, hoarseness, or airway obstruction
- ⚠ History of TB exposure, HIV or immunosuppression
- ⚠ Chest pain with cough (pleuritic or retrosternal)

∏ Haemoptysis:
- ❖ **Implications/Diagnoses:** Lung cancer, PE, TB, Bronchiectasis.
- ❖ **Investigations:** CXR, CT chest, bronchoscopy + biopsy, sputum cytology, CTPA, D-dimer, ECG, ABG, sputum AFB, GeneXpert PCR, HRCT chest, sputum culture.

∏ Unintentional weight loss, anorexia, night sweats:
- ❖ **Implications/Diagnoses:** Lung cancer, TB, Lymphoma, Fungal infections.
- ❖ **Investigations:** CXR, CT chest, PET-CT, bronchoscopy, sputum AFB, QuantiFERON Gold, culture, LDH, excisional node biopsy, fungal serology, sputum culture.

∏ Persistent cough > 8 weeks, not improving:
- **Implications/Diagnoses:** Lung cancer, TB, Interstitial Lung disease, Asthma/COPD, GORD.
- **Implications:** CXR, CT chest, bronchoscopy, sputum AFB, GeneXpert PCR, HRCT chest, PFTs, autoimmune screen, spirometry with reversibility, peak flow diary, 24-hr esophageal pH monitoring, endoscopy.

∏ Smoking history (>40yrs) with new/changing cough:
- **Implications/Diagnoses:** Lung cancer, COPD exacerbations.
- **Investigations:** CXR, CT chest, PET-CT, bronchoscopy ± biopsy, spirometry, ABG.

∏ Dyspnoea, pleuritic chest pain, haemoptysis (classic PE triad):
- **Implications:** PE.
- **Investigations:** Wells score, D-dimer, CTPA, ECG, V/Q scan.

∏ Fever, rigors, productive purulent sputum, pleuritic pain:
- **Implications/Diagnoses:** Pneumonia, Lung abscess/empyema, TB.
- **Investigations:** CXR, sputum & blood cultures, CRP, CT chest, pleural fluid aspiration, sputum AFB, GeneXpert PCR.

∏ Clubbing or chronic purulent sputum production:
- **Implications/Diagnoses:** Bronchiectasis, cystic fibrosis, Lung abscess.
- **Investigations:** HRCT chest, sputum culture, PFTs, sweat chloride test, CFTR genetic testing, CT chest.

∏ Stridor, hoarseness, or airway obstruction:
- **Implications/Diagnoses:** Laryngeal cancer, foreign body aspiration, mediastinal mass, Epiglottis.

- **Investigations:** Laryngoscopy with biopsy, CT/MRI neck & chest, CXR, CT airway, bronchoscopy, mediastinoscopy, EBUS, nasoendoscopy.

∏ History of TB exposure, HIV or immunosuppression:
- **Implications/Diagnoses:** TB, PCP pneumonia, fungal infections.
- **Investigations:** CXR, sputum AFB, GeneXpert PCR, culture, CT chest, sputum/BAL for PCP PCR, LDH, fungal serology, sputum or BAL culture.

∏ Chest pain with cough (pleuritic or retrosternal):
- **Implications/Diagnoses:** PE, Pneumonia, Pericarditis, Lung cancer invasion.
- **Investigations:** CTPA, D-dimer, ECG, CXR, sputum culture, blood cultures, troponin, echo, CT chest, PET-CT, biopsy.

🗝 Key points:
- First-line for any cough red flag = CXR + baseline bloods(FBC, CRP, UEC, LFTs).
- Haemoptysis, weight loss, smoking history or > 8 weeks persistent cough warrants urgent 2 weeks referral for suspected cancer.
- TB suspicion – sputum AFB × 3 + GeneXpert + CXR.
- Acute cough most common causes are URTI, postnasal drip, COPD exacerbations, and Pneumonia.
- Occult gastroesophageal reflux disease is a overlooked cause.

ABC approach to Cough (evaluation + workup):

A — Assessment and immediate threats (rule out "can't miss")

Triage severity

- **Obs/NEWS2, SpO$_2$**, RR, HR, BP, temp; assess work of breathing.
- Give **O$_2$ if hypoxic**, sit up, bronchodilator if severe wheeze.

Immediate threats + clues + urgent actions

- **Airway compromise** (stridor, drooling, voice change, anaphylaxis) → ABCDE, adrenaline if anaphylaxis, urgent senior/ENT/anaesthetics.
- **Severe asthma/COPD** (silent chest, exhaustion, SpO$_2$ low) → nebs, steroids, ABG/VBG, consider NIV/ITU.
- **Pneumonia / sepsis** (fever, pleuritic pain, rigors, hypotension) → sepsis bundle, blood cultures, IV antibiotics, CXR.
- **Pulmonary embolism** (pleuritic pain, tachycardia, hypoxia, syncope, leg swelling) → risk stratify, D-dimer if appropriate, **CTPA** if indicated.
- **ACS/HF** (chest pain, orthopnoea, oedema, crackles) → ECG, troponin if ACS, BNP if HF suspected, CXR.
- **Massive haemoptysis** → resus, protect airway, urgent CT/bronchoscopy pathway.
- **TB / malignancy red flags** (weight loss, night sweats, persistent cough, haemoptysis) → isolate if TB risk; urgent imaging/referral.

B — Bedside assessment (focused history and exam)

Focused history

- **Duration:** acute <3w / subacute 3–8w / chronic >8w
- **Type:** dry vs productive; sputum volume/colour; **haemoptysis**
- **Associated:** fever, dyspnoea, wheeze, chest pain, weight loss, night sweats, reflux/heartburn, post-nasal drip/rhinitis, voice change
- **Triggers:** exercise, cold air, allergens, lying flat, meals
- **Exposures:** smoking/vaping, occupation (dust/chemicals), travel, TB contacts, pets/mould
- **PMH:** asthma/COPD, HF, bronchiectasis, ILD, immunosuppression, aspiration risk (stroke/dysphagia)
- **Meds: ACE-inhibitor** (common), beta-blockers, inhalers (technique/adherence)

Focused exam

- **Vitals** (SpO_2 key), fever, respiratory distress, cyanosis
- **ENT:** nasal mucosa, post-nasal drip, sinus tenderness, throat
- **Chest:** wheeze (asthma/COPD), focal crackles/bronchial breathing (pneumonia), widespread crackles (HF/ILD), reduced breath sounds (effusion/pneumothorax)
- **CVS:** JVP, oedema, displaced apex, murmurs
- **Peripheral:** calf swelling (DVT), clubbing (malignancy/ILD/bronchiectasis)

C- Core investigations (workup)

Baseline (most patients with significant/persistent cough)

- **CXR** (especially >3 weeks, abnormal exam, smokers, systemic symptoms, haemoptysis)
- **FBC, U&E, CRP** (infection/inflammation; anaemia)
- **ECG** if chest pain/tachycardia or HF/PE consideration
- **Pulse oximetry** ± **ABG/VBG** if hypoxic, severe COPD/asthma, or drowsy

If productive / infection suspected

- **Sputum culture** (and sensitivity) if purulent, severe, recurrent, or immunosuppressed
- **Blood cultures** if febrile/septic
- Viral testing (seasonal/outbreak setting)

If asthma/COPD suspected

- **Spirometry** (with bronchodilator reversibility if asthma)
- **Peak flow diary** (variability)
- **FeNO** / eosinophils if available (eosinophilic airway disease)

If PE suspected

- Use local pathway (e.g., Wells/PERC as applicable):
  - **D-dimer** if low/intermediate risk
  - **CTPA** (or V/Q if appropriate) if indicated

If HF suspected

- **BNP/NT-proBNP** (per local pathway) ± **echo**
- CXR for congestion/effusions

If TB or malignancy features

- TB: **IGRA ± sputum AFB** (3 samples) and isolation if high suspicion
- **CT chest** if abnormal CXR or persistent unexplained cough / weight loss / haemoptysis
- Consider urgent (2-week) referral per local criteria

Mnemonic- Causes of chronic cough: **COUGH IT UP**

👉 Covers common and serious causes

C – COPD / Chronic bronchitis (smoker's cough)

O – Obstructive airway 🚩
- Asthma, bronchiectasis
- Foreign body 🚩

U – Upper airway
- Post-nasal drip, rhinitis, sinusitis

G – GERD / GORD
- Reflux-related cough

H – Heart failure 🚩
- Pulmonary oedema, "cardiac asthma"

I – Infection
- Acute bronchitis, pneumonia 🚩, TB 🚩

T – Tumour 🚩
- Lung cancer, mediastinal mass

U – Unusual interstitial disease
- Pulmonary fibrosis, sarcoidosis

P – Pulmonary embolism 🚩
- Haemoptysis, pleuritic pain, SOB

Mnemonic for Red Flags in Cough: "CRISIS"

👉 The features that make you stop and think "serious"

C – Coughing blood (haemoptysis → cancer, TB, PE)

R – Recurrent / persistent >8 weeks despite treatment

I – Immunosuppressed (HIV, chemo, transplant → TB, fungal, PCP)

S – Systemic features (fever, night sweats, weight loss → TB, malignancy)

I – Increasing breathlessness or hypoxia (PE, pneumonia, HF, fibrosis)

S – Smoker / high-risk occupation with new cough (lung cancer)

✅ How to remember:

- **"COUGH IT UP"** → think of coughing something up → causes.
- **"CRISIS"** → think: if these appear with cough, it's a crisis / red flag.

Confusion

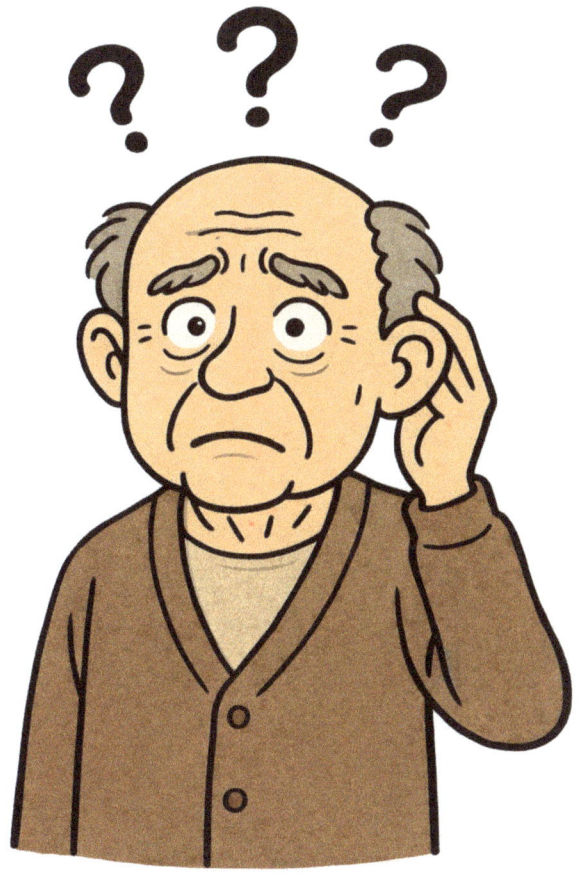

▶ Red Flags: Confusion

- ⚠ Sudden onset confusion(<hours-days)
- ⚠ Headache, meningism, photophobia, fever
- ⚠ History of trauma or fall (esp. on anticoagulants)
- ⚠ Focal neurological deficit
- ⚠ Severe agitation, fluctuating consciousness, disorientation
- ⚠ Hypotension, tachycardia, fever, rigors
- ⚠ Hypoglycaemia/Hyperglcaemia
- ⚠ Polyuria, dehydration, polydipsia, recent illness
- ⚠ History of alcohol misuse/withdrawal, poor nutrition
- ⚠ Immunosuppressed, HIV, recent travel
- ⚠ New medication or drug withdrawal
- ⚠ Elderly, fluctuating course, acute hospitalisation

∏ Sudden onset confusion:
- ❖ **Implications/Diagnoses:** Stroke, intracranial haemorrhage, seizure/post-ictal, acute infection/sepsis.
- ❖ **Investigations:** FBC, UEC, CRP, glucose, ECG, CT/MRI brain, EEG.

∏ Headache, meningism, photophobia, fever:
- ❖ **Implications/Diagnoses:** Meningitis, encephalitis, subarachnoid haemorrhage.
- ❖ **Investigations:** CT brain, LP(after excluding raised ICP), blood cultures, viral PCR, CRP/ESR.

∏ History of trauma or fall (esp. on anticoagulants):

- **Implications/Diagnoses:** Subdural/epidural haematoma, intracranial bleed.
- **Implications/Diagnoses:** coagulation profile, anticoagulation levels, CT head.

∏ Focal neurological deficit (weakness, dysphasia, visual loss, ataxia):

- **Implications/Diagnoses:** Stroke/TIA, brain tumour, space-occupying lesion.
- **Implications/Diagnoses:** CT/MRI brain, carotid doppler, echocardiogram.

∏ Severe agitation, fluctuating, consciousness, disorientation:

- **Implications/Diagnoses:** Delerium (often infection, metabolic, drug, or infection).
- **Investigations:** FBC, UEC, glucose, LFT, calcium, TFT, B12/folate, urine dip/MSU, CT head.

∏ Hypotension, tachycardia, fever, rigors:

- **Implications/Diagnoses:** Sepsis (urosepsis, pneumonia, endocarditis).
- **Investigations:** sepsis 6- blood cultures, urine culture, CXR, lactate, CRP, ECG.

∏ Hypoglycaemia/Hyperglycaemia:

- **Implications/Diagnoses:** Hypoglycaemia, DKA, HHS.
- **Investigations:** Capillary glucose, ABG (ketones, acidosis), UEC, osmolality.

∏ Polyuria, dehydration, polydipsia, recent illness:

- **Implications/Diagnoses:** Electrolyte disturbance, renal failure.
- **Investigations:** UEC, calcium, osmolality, ABG, ECG.

∏ History of alcohol misuse/withdrawal, poor nutrition:
* **Implications/Diagnoses:** Wernicke's encephalopathy, alcohol withdrawal delirium.
* **Investigations:** Neuro exam, LFT, MCV, CT head.

∏ Immunosuppressed, HIV, recent travel:
* **Implications/Diagnoses:** Opportunistic CNS infections (cryptococcus, toxoplasmosis), malaria, encephalitis.
* **Investigations:** HIV screen, malaria film, blood cultures, CT/MRI brain , LP (if no contraindications).

∏ New medication or drug withdrawal:
* **Implications/Diagnoses:** Anticholinergic toxicity, opioid/benzo withdrawal, serotonin syndrome, neuroleptic malignant syndrome.
* **Investigations:** Medication review, CK, TFT, UEC, toxicology screen.

∏ Elderly, fluctuating course, acute hospitalisation:
* **Implications/Diagnoses:** Delerium superimposed on dementia.
* **Investigations:** FBC, UEC, LFT, glucose, urinalysis, CXR.

🗝 Key points:
- Always check capillary glucose first in any confused patient and it is rapidly reversible.
- ABG helps assess hypoxia, hypercapnia and metabolic abnormalities.
- Confusion in elderly = infection until proven otherwise (especially pneumonia, UTI).
- Getting collateral history from family/carers is vital to establish baseline cognition.

- Consider CT head if no obvious cause on infection screen, exam.

ABC approach to Confusion (evaluation + workup):

A — Assessment and immediate threats

1) Rapid severity check (ABCDE + vitals)
- **Obs/NEWS2, SpO$_2$**, RR, HR, BP, temp, glucose
- Look for **hypoxia, hypotension, fever, hypoglycaemia, hypercapnia**
- Ensure safety: falls risk, remove hazards, 1:1 if needed

2) Immediate threats to treat now (with first actions)
- **Hypoglycaemia** → check capillary glucose, give glucose
- **Hypoxia / respiratory failure** → oxygen, ABG/VBG if needed
- **Sepsis** (esp. pneumonia/UTI/abdominal) → sepsis bundle, cultures, antibiotics, fluids
- **Stroke / ICH** (new focal deficit, severe headache, anticoagulation, reduced GCS) → urgent CT head + stroke/neurology pathway
- **Meningitis/encephalitis** (fever, neck stiffness, photophobia, seizures, rash) → urgent antibiotics/acyclovir per pathway + LP when safe
- **Toxicology/overdose** (opioids, benzos, alcohol withdrawal, CO exposure) → targeted antidotes (e.g., naloxone), supportive care
- **Hypercapnia** (COPD, sedatives) → ABG, NIV if indicated

- **Seizure / non-convulsive status** (fluctuating confusion, subtle twitching) → urgent senior/EEG pathway
- **Raised ICP** (vomiting, papilloedema, focal signs) → urgent imaging; avoid LP until excluded
- **Severe agitation/violence** risking harm → de-escalation first; short-term sedation per local policy

B — Bedside assessment (focused history and exam)

Focused history (from patient, family, carers, notes)

- **Onset & course:** acute vs chronic, fluctuating (delirium), time last seen well
- **Baseline cognition/function:** dementia? independence? sensory impairment?
- **Precipitants:** infection symptoms, pain, constipation/urinary retention, dehydration, sleep deprivation
- **Drugs/substances:** new meds, **anticholinergics**, opioids, benzos, steroids; alcohol intake/withdrawal; recreational drugs
- **Medical risks:** recent surgery, ICU, falls/head injury, anticoagulation, CKD/liver disease
- **Neuro symptoms:** headache, seizures, focal weakness, speech/vision change
- **Exposure:** CO (heaters), toxins, recent travel, sick contacts

Focused exam

- **Mental status:** attention (months backward), arousal, hallucinations, agitation vs hypoactive
- **Neuro:** pupils, limb power, speech, gait (if safe), meningism, asterixis

- **General:** hydration, fever, rash, jaundice, signs of trauma
- **Chest/heart/abdomen:** pneumonia/HF clues; abdominal tenderness
- **Bladder/bowel:** suprapubic fullness, **constipation**
- **Bedside tests:** capillary glucose, bladder scan if retention suspected

C- Core investigations (workup)

Baseline for most acute confusion (especially suspected delirium)

- **Bloods:** FBC, U&E/creatinine, CRP, LFT, **calcium**, glucose, magnesium, TFT (if unclear), B12/folate if chronic
- **Infection screen:** urinalysis ± culture (if symptomatic), **CXR** if respiratory features, blood cultures if febrile/septic
- **ECG** (arrhythmia, QTc—important if using antipsychotics)
- **ABG/VBG** if hypoxic, COPD, drowsy, or concern for hypercapnia
- **Medication review** and drug levels where relevant (e.g., lithium, digoxin)

Targeted tests (based on clues)

- **CT head if:** head injury/fall, anticoagulated, focal neurology, seizure, reduced GCS, persistent unexplained acute confusion
- **Lumbar puncture** if meningitis/encephalitis suspected **after** imaging if indicated

- **Toxicology:** ethanol level, paracetamol/salicylate (as appropriate), urine drug screen if relevant
- **Thiamine** (give before glucose in suspected Wernicke's)
- **EEG** if suspected non-convulsive status
- **TSH, cortisol** if endocrine cause suspected (e.g., adrenal crisis features)
- **Ammonia** if severe liver disease/encephalopathy suspected

Mnemonic for causes of Delerium: DELIRIUM

- **D** Drugs
- **E** Epilepsy/electrolyte imbalance
- **L** Liver failure/low oxygen (MI, PE)
- **I** Infections
- **R** Retention (urine, faecal)
- **I** Intracranial -stroke, TIA, traumatic head injury
- **U** Uremia
- **M** Metabolic- anaemia, Hypoglycaemia, endocrine problems, electrolyte abnormalities.

Mnemonics for causes of Delerium: PINCH ME

- **P** Pain
- **I** Infection
- **N** Nutrition
- **C** Constipation
- **H** Hydration
- **M** Medications
- **E** Environment

Mnemonic for red flags of delirium: "RED FLAG"

R – Recent trauma / fall with head injury (subdural, ICH)

E – Evidence of infection (pneumonia, UTI, meningitis, sepsis)

D – Dehydration / severe metabolic upset (Na, Ca, glucose extremes, renal/hepatic failure)

F – Focal neurology / new seizures (stroke, SOL, encephalitis)

L – Low oxygen / hypoxia (PE, COPD, pneumonia)

A – Acute cardiac event (MI, arrhythmia, shock, heart failure)

G – Gross cognitive decline or rapid deterioration (possible malignancy, rapidly progressive dementia, encephalitis)

Common drugs causing or worsening delirium : 8As.

Antibiotics	quinolones, macrolides, cephalosporins.
Antidepressants	TCA, SSRI
Anticholinergic	TCA, oxybutynin
Anti-pain/anxiolytics	Opioid, Benzodiazepines.
Anti-immune	Steroids
Anti-Parkinson	all types
Antipsychotics	prochorpromazine
Anticonvulsants	phenytoin

Diarrhea

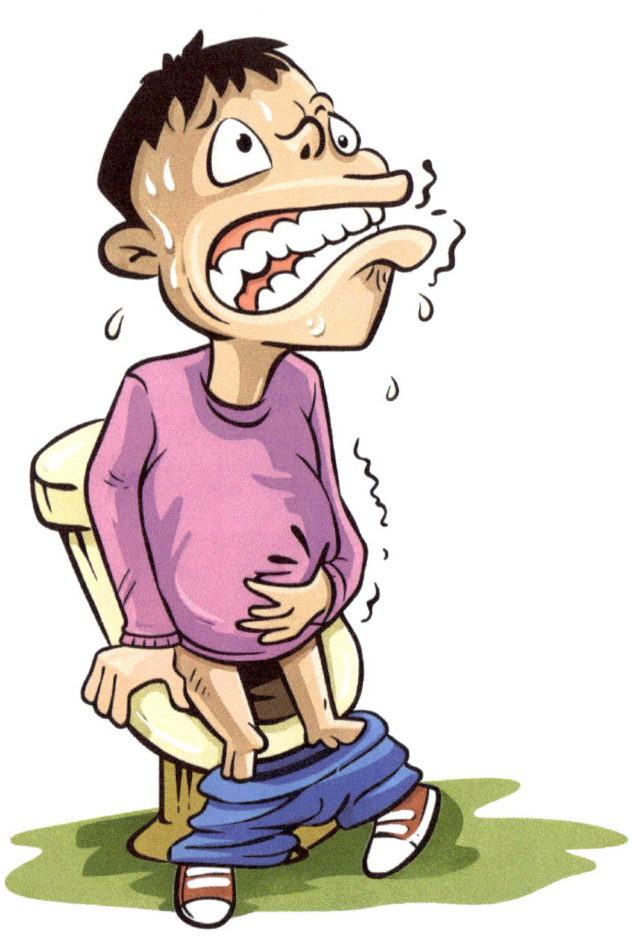

▶ Red Flags: Diarrhea

- ⚠ Blood or mucus in stool (haematochezia/melaena)
- ⚠ Unintentional weight loss
- ⚠ Nocturnal diarrhea
- ⚠ Persistent diarrhea > 4 weeks
- ⚠ Family history of colorectal cancer/IBD
- ⚠ Anaemia
- ⚠ Fever and systemic illness
- ⚠ Severe abdominal pain, Peritonism or distension
- ⚠ Age>50 with new-onset diarrhea
- ⚠ Recent hospitalization/antibiotics use
- ⚠ Dehydration/shock (Hypotension, tachycardia)
- ⚠ Steatorrhea
- ⚠ Fever>38.5 C, raised inflammatory markers
- ⚠ Immunosuppressed (HIV, chemotherapy)
- ⚠ Acidosis on ABG, raised Lactate

∏ Blood or mucus in stool:
- ❖ **Implications/Diagnoses:** IBD, Colorectal cancer, infectious colitis, ischaemic colitis.
- ❖ **Investigations:** Colonoscopy with biopsy, CT colonography, CT angiogram, CRP, faecal calprotectin, stool culture, ova/cyst/parasites (OCP), C.diff toxin.

∏ Unintentional weight loss:
- ❖ **Implications/Diagnoses:** Malignancy, IBD, Coeliac disease.
- ❖ **Investigations:** Colonoscopy, CT colonography, CT abdomen/pelvis, faecal calprotectin, coeliac serology(tTG, IgA), duodenal biopsy.

∏ Nocturnal diarrhea:
- ❖ **Implications/Diagnoses:** IBD, Infection, Microscopic colitis.
- ❖ **Investigations:** Colonoscopy with biopsy, faecal calprotectin, stool cultures, C-diff toxin, OCP (ova, cyst and parasite).

∏ Persistent diarrhea > 4 weeks:
- ❖ **Implications/Diagnoses:** Chronic infection(Giardia, TB), IBD, Malabsorption, Endocrine.
- ❖ **Investigations:** Stool OCP/PCR, stool antigen, colonoscopy with IBD, Coeliac serology, faecal elastase, vitamin levels, TFTs, ACTH, VIP, gastrin.

∏ Family history of colorectal cancer/IBD:
- ❖ **Implications/Diagnoses:** Colorectal cancer, IBD,
- ❖ **Investigations:** colonoscopy ± genetic testing (HNPCC/FAP), FOB/FIT, faecal calprotectin.

∏ Anaemia:
- ❖ **Implications/Diagnoses:** Chronic blood loss (colorectal cancer, IBD), Malabsorption (coeliac, pancreatic insufficiency).
- ❖ **Investigations:** FBC, iron studies, colonoscopy, upper GI endoscopy, coeliac serology, faecal elastase, vitamin B12/folate.

∏ Fever & systemic illnesses:
- ❖ **Implications/Diagnoses:** severe infection, IBD flare, sepsis.
- ❖ **Investigations:** stool cultures, C-diff toxin PCR, blood cultures, CRP, faecal calprotectin, colonoscopy(if stable), lactate, CT abdomen (perforation/abscess if suspected).

∏ Severe abdominal pain/distension:

- **Implications/Diagnoses:** Obstruction, Toxic megacolon, Ischaemic colitis.
- **Investigations:** AXR, CT abdomen/pelvis, colonoscopy (if stable), CT angiogram.

∏ Age>50 with new-onset diarrhea:

- **Implications/Diagnoses:** Colorectal cancer, Microscopic colitis, IBD.
- **Investigations:** Colonoscopy ± biopsy, CT colonography, faecal calprotectin.

∏ Recent hospitalization/antibiotics:

- **Implications/Diagnoses:** C-difficile colitis.
- **Investigations:** stool toxin PCR, FBC, UEC, flexible sigmoidoscopy if severe.

∏ Dehydration/shock:

- **Implications/Diagnoses:** severe acute diarrhea(cholera, gastroenteritis), melaena (GI bleed).
- **Investigations:** FBC, UEC, ABG, stool cultures, blood cultures, lactate, OGD.

∏ Steatorrheas:

- **Implications/Diagnoses:** Chronic pancreatitis, coeliac disease, bile salt malabsorption.
- **Investigations:** faecal elastase, MRI/CT pancreas, coeliac serology, duodenal biopsy, SeHCAT test.

∏ Fever> 38.5 , raised inflammatory markers:

- **Implications/Diagnoses:** Infectious colitis, systemic infection.
- **Investigations:** FBC, CRP, stool culture, blood culture.

⌂ Immunosuppressed (HIV, chemotherapy):

* **Implications/Diagnoses:** opportunistic infections(CMV, Cryptosporidium).
* **Investigations:** stool PCR panel, colonoscopy with biopsy, HIV viral load/CD4 count.

⌂ Acidosis on ABG, raised Lactate:

* **Implications/Diagnoses:** Mesenteric ischaemia
* **Investigations:** ABG, CT angiogram, CT abdomen with contrast.
* Look for AF, embolic source.

🗝 Key points:

- Red flag point away from IBS(functional cause) and toward organic pathology(infection, IBD, cancer, malabsorption, ischaemia).
- The most common causes of acute diarrhea -Gastroenteritis(typically viral), Food poisoning.
- The most common causes of chronic diarrhea-Functional disorders, IBD, others(drugs, malabsorption, drugs).
- Acute, watery diarrhea in an otherwise healthy person is likely to be of infectious etiology-check travel history, contaminated food, outbreak with a point-source.
- Acute bloody diarrhea in an otherwise healthy person suggests an enteroinvasive infection. Ischaemic colitis and Diverticular bleeding also present with acute bloody diarrhea.
- Recurrent bouts of bloody diarrhea in a younger person suggests Inflammatory bowel disease.

ABC approach to Diarrhoea (evaluation + workup):

A — Assessment and immediate threats

Rapid severity check

- Obs/NEWS2, **hydration status**, mental state, urine output, postural BP, pain.
- Look for **shock**, severe dehydration, sepsis.

Immediate threats / red flags (urgent same-day assessment)

- **Severe dehydration/shock:** hypotension, tachycardia, syncope, oliguria
- **Sepsis/toxic appearance** or high fever
- **Blood/mucus** in stool, severe abdominal pain, peritonism
- **Suspected acute abdomen:** guarding/rebound, distension, absent bowel sounds
- **Severe/profuse diarrhoea** (>6/day) or unable to maintain oral intake
- **Immunosuppressed**, frail elderly, significant comorbidity
- **Recent antibiotics / recent admission → C. difficile risk**
- **Recent travel**, outbreak exposure, unsafe water/food
- **Persistent diarrhoea >14 days**, weight loss, nocturnal symptoms
- **Pregnancy** (dehydration risk; consider specific causes)

Immediate actions if red flags present

- IV access, **fluids**, correct electrolytes, strict input/output
- Stool isolation if infectious suspected (especially **suspected C. diff**)

- Early senior/surgical review if peritonism/obstruction/megacolon concern

B — Bedside assessment (focused history and exam)

Focused history

- **Duration:** acute (<14 days) vs persistent (14–28 days) vs chronic (>4 weeks)
- **Character:** watery vs bloody vs fatty/greasy; volume; nocturnal symptoms; urgency/tenesmus
- **Associated symptoms:** fever, vomiting, abdominal pain, weight loss, rash, arthralgia
- **Exposures:** travel, sick contacts, food (undercooked poultry/eggs/seafood), unpasteurised dairy, camping/streams
- **Recent antibiotics**, PPIs, laxatives; recent hospital/care home exposure
- **PMH:** IBD, IBS, coeliac, pancreatitis, thyroid disease, diabetes, immunosuppression
- **Meds:** metformin, magnesium, antibiotics, chemotherapy, SSRIs, NSAIDs
- **Dehydration clues:** thirst, dizziness, reduced urine; blood in stool amount
- **Risk of complications:** frailty, CKD, heart failure (fluid balance)

Focused exam

- **General:** hydration (mucosa, skin turgor), capillary refill, postural drop
- **Vitals:** temp, HR, BP, RR, SpO_2

- **Abdominal:** tenderness, guarding/rebound, masses, distension
- **PR exam** if blood, severe pain, or diagnostic uncertainty
- Consider signs of **systemic disease** (rash, arthritis, thyrotoxicosis)

C- Core investigations (workup)

Baseline (moderate–severe, frail, comorbid, or admitted patients)

- **FBC** (anaemia, leukocytosis), **U&E/creatinine** (AKI), **CRP**
- **LFTs**, **magnesium, calcium** (if severe/prolonged)
- **VBG/ABG + lactate** if shock/sepsis concern

Stool tests (send based on scenario)

- **Stool culture/PCR** (acute infectious features: fever, blood, severe illness, outbreak, travel)
- **C. difficile toxin/PCR if recent antibiotics or healthcare exposure** or unexplained diarrhoea in hospital
- **Ova, cysts & parasites / Giardia** if travel, camping, prolonged watery diarrhoea
- **Faecal calprotectin** if chronic diarrhoea with inflammatory features (suspected IBD)

Other targeted tests

- **Blood cultures** if febrile/septic
- **Pregnancy test** where relevant
- **Coeliac screen** (tTG-IgA + total IgA) if chronic diarrhoea/weight loss

- **TSH** if chronic diarrhoea with hyperthyroid symptoms
- **Lipase/amylase** if pancreatic features; consider malabsorption workup if fatty stools

Imaging / escalation

- **CT abdomen/pelvis** if severe abdominal pain, peritonism, suspected colitis complications, obstruction, or toxic megacolon
- **Flexible sigmoidoscopy/colonoscopy** if suspected IBD, persistent bloody diarrhoea, or red flags (as per pathway)

📋 Mnemonic - Causes of Diarrhea: **DIARRHOEA**

👉 Covers **common** + **serious causes**

D – Drugs
- Antibiotics (C. diff 🚩), laxatives, chemotherapy, metformin

I – Infection
- Viral gastroenteritis, bacterial (Salmonella, Shigella, Campylobacter), parasitic (Giardia, Entamoeba)

A – Alcohol / Abuse
- Alcohol excess, stimulant laxative abuse

R – Rectal disease
- Proctitis, colorectal cancer 🚩

R – Reduced absorption (malabsorption)
- Coeliac disease, pancreatic insufficiency, bile salt malabsorption

H – Hormonal / Endocrine
- Hyperthyroidism, Addison's disease 🚩, VIPoma

O – Obstruction overflow
- Constipation with overflow diarrhoea

E – Enteropathy inflammatory
- IBD (Crohn's, UC 🚩), microscopic colitis

A – Anxiety / functional
- IBS, stress-related

Mnemonic for Red Flags in Diarrhoea: "STOOL RED"

👉 Think: if stool is RED, be alert

S – Severe dehydration / shock
- Hypotension, tachycardia, acute kidney injury

T – Tenesmus / nocturnal symptoms
- Suggests IBD or malignancy

O – Ongoing >6 weeks (chronic)
- Cancer, malabsorption, endocrine

O – Old age (>50) with new symptoms
- Colorectal cancer risk

L – Large-volume blood / melaena
- IBD flare, ischaemic colitis, cancer

R – Recent antibiotics / hospitalisation
- C. difficile infection

E – Evidence of systemic illness
- Weight loss, fever, night sweats, cachexia

D – Dangerous comorbidities / immunosuppression
- HIV, chemo, transplant, neutropenia

✅ **How to remember**
- **"DIARRHOEA"** → the broad causes.
- **"STOOL RED"** → the danger signs (red flags).

Diplopia

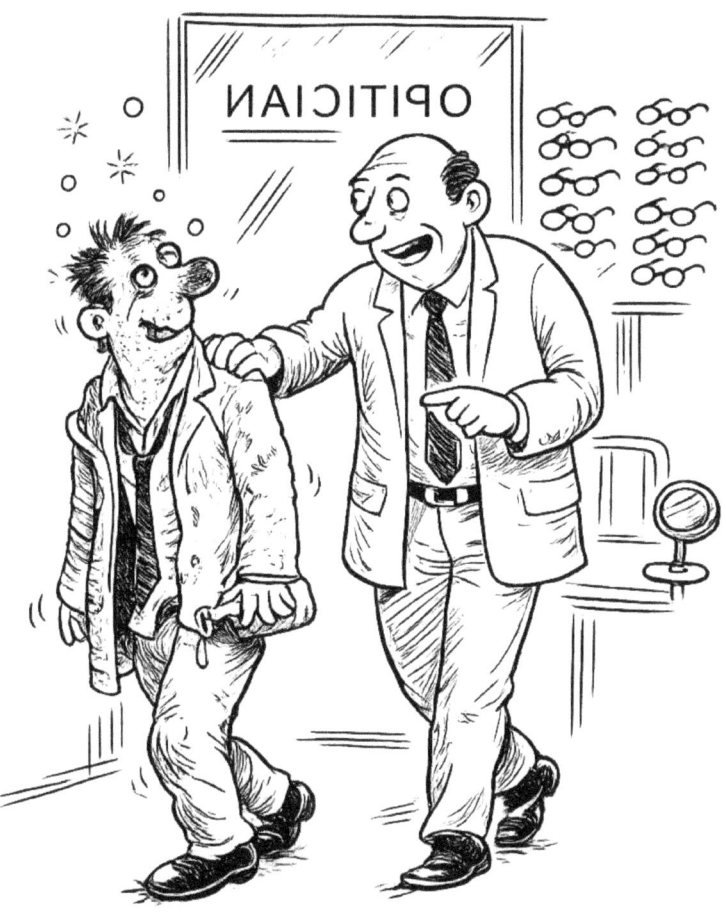

"Come back when you're sober, and we'll see if you still have that double vision."

⚑ Red Flags: Diplopia

- ⚠ **Acute onset diplopia (sudden, hours to days)**
- ⚠ **Diplopia with headache, severe eye pain, or periorbital swelling**
- ⚠ **Diplopia with pupillary involvement (fixed dilated pupil in CN 3rd palsy)**
- ⚠ **Diplopia with other neurological deficits (weakness, numbness, ataxia, dysarthria, dysphagia)**
- ⚠ **Diplopia with fluctuating muscle weakness or ptosis**
- ⚠ **Diplopia with proptosis, lid lag, or thyroid signs**
- ⚠ **Diplopia with trauma history**
- ⚠ **Diplopia with systemic symptoms (fever, weight loss, night sweats, jaw claudication, scalp tenderness)**
- ⚠ **Multiple cranial nerve deficits**

Acute onset diplopia (sudden, hours to days):
- ❖ **Implications/Diagnoses:** Vascular or neurological emergency- Stroke/TIA, aneurysm, giant cell arteritis (GCA), raised ICP.
- ❖ **Investigations:** CT/MRI brain, urgent CTA/MRA brain, carotid doppler, ECG, glucose, cholesterol, ESR, CRP, temporal artery biopsy.

Diplopia with headache, severe eye pain, or periorbital swelling:
- ❖ **Implications/Diagnoses:** Neurological, vascular, or orbital pathology-cavernous sinus thrombosis, carotid-cavernous fistula, orbital cellulitis, aneurysm.

- ❖ **Investigations:** MRI/MRV brain & orbits, CT orbit with contrast, blood cultures, Lumbar puncture.

Diplopia with pupillary involvement (fixed dilated pupil in CN 3rd palsy):

- ❖ **Implications/Diagnoses:** Posterior communicating artery aneurysm-Aneurysmal third nerve palsy.
- ❖ **Investigations:** Urgent CTA/MRA, MRI brain/orbits.

Diplopia with other neurological deficits (weakness, numbness, ataxia, dysarthria, dysphagia):

- ❖ **Implications/Diagnoses:** brainstem or demyelinating disease-stroke, multiple sclerosis, brainstem tumour.
- ❖ **Investigations:** MRI brain with orbits with contrast, CSF analysis, stroke workup-CT/MRI, carotid doppler, ECG, echo.

Diplopia with fluctuating muscle weakness or ptosis:

- ❖ **Implications/Diagnoses:** Neuromuscular junction disorder-Myasthenia gravis.
- ❖ **Investigations:** AChR and MuSK antibodies, Repetitive nerve stimulation/EMG, CT/MRU chest(thymoma screening).

Diplopia with proptosis, lid lag, or thyroid signs:

- ❖ **Implications/Diagnoses:** Endocrine/autoimmune orbital disease-Thyroid eye disease (Grave/s orbitopathy).
- ❖ **Investigations:** TFTs, thyroid antibodies, orbital CT/MRI (extraocular muscle enlargement).

Diplopia with trauma history:

- ❖ **Implications/Diagnoses:** orbital fracture, extraocular muscle entrapment, traumatic CN palsy 3rd, 4th, 6th.
- ❖ **Investigations:** CT orbit/facial bones, ophthalmology slit-lamp exam.

∏ Diplopia with systemic symptoms (fever, weight loss, night sweats, jaw claudication, scalp tenderness):

- ❖ **Implications/Diagnoses:** vasculitis or malignancy- GCA, Lymphoma, orbital tumour.
- ❖ **Investigations:** ESR, CRP, temporal artery biopsy(GCA), CT/MRI orbit/brain, biopsy of orbital lesion if mass suspected.

∏ Multiple cranial nerve deficits:

- ❖ **Implications/Diagnoses:** Neurological disorder- primary malignancy/metastasis, compression from tumor, stroke, autoimmune-Lupus, GBS.
- ❖ **Investigations:** CT/MRI brain, stroke screen, autoimmune screen.

🗝 Key points:

- Sudden -onset diplopia, painful diplopia, pupillary involvement, or associated neuro deficits are red flags requiring urgent imaging (MRI/CT/CTA).
- All diplopia with systemic features- investigate for vasculitis, malignancy, infection.
- Monocular diplopia is due to distortion of light transmission through the eye to the retina. The most common causes are- Cataract, corneal shape problems such as keratoconus, Uncorrected refractive errors usually astigmatism. Dislocated lens and corneal scarring are other causes.
- Binocular diplopia is due to disconjugate alignment of the eyes. The most common causes are- Cranial nerve 3rd, 4th, or 6th palsy, Myasthenia gravis, orbital infiltration.

ABC approach to Diplopia (evaluation + workup):

A — Assessment and immediate threats

1) First confirm this is true diplopia
- Ask: **Does it disappear when either eye is closed?**
  - **Yes** → **binocular diplopia** (misalignment; neuro/ocular motor causes; potentially urgent)
  - **No** → **monocular diplopia** (usually ocular/refractive; less often life-threatening)

2) Rapid red flags (urgent same-day / ED / stroke pathway)
- **Brainstem stroke/TIA:** sudden onset + **focal neuro deficits** (dysarthria, ataxia, vertigo, hemiparesis, facial numbness)
- **Aneurysm / compressive 3rd nerve palsy: ptosis + "down and out" eye + dilated pupil** or severe headache
- **Giant cell arteritis (age ≥50):** new headache, scalp tenderness, jaw claudication, visual symptoms
- **Cavernous sinus/orbital apex pathology:** diplopia + **severe headache, proptosis**, chemosis, reduced corneal sensation, multiple CN palsies
- **Raised ICP:** headache worse on waking, vomiting, papilloedema
- **Meningitis/encephalitis:** fever, neck stiffness, photophobia, altered consciousness
- **Trauma** (orbital fracture, head injury), **anticoagulated + head injury**
- **Myasthenic crisis / respiratory compromise** (fatigable bulbar symptoms, breathlessness)

Immediate actions if red flags
- Obs/NEWS2, glucose if altered, analgesia/antiemetic
- **Urgent neuro-ophthalmic assessment**
- **Stroke/ICH pathway** if acute focal neurology
- **Urgent CT/CTA or MRI/MRA** depending on scenario (see workup)
- If suspected **GCA:** start **high-dose steroids immediately** + urgent ESR/CRP and ophthalmology/rheum pathway

B — Bedside assessment (focused history and exam)

Focused history
- **Onset:** sudden vs gradual; constant vs intermittent; duration; progression
- **Binocular vs monocular** (cover test history)
- **Direction:** horizontal/vertical/oblique; worse in which gaze? distance vs near?
- **Associated symptoms:**
  - Ptosis, anisocoria, eye pain, headache
  - Vertigo, ataxia, dysarthria, numbness/weakness
  - Thyroid symptoms (grittiness, lid retraction), orbital pain
  - Fatigability (worse late day), chewing/swallowing issues (myasthenia)
- **Risk factors:** vascular (DM/HTN), smoking, AF, migraine, trauma
- **Systemic:** recent infection, autoimmune disease, cancer history
- **Medications/toxins:** alcohol, sedatives (less commonly direct cause, more confounders)

Focused exam (high-yield)

1) Quick eye screening

- **Visual acuity** (each eye), colour vision (red desaturation), visual fields
- Inspect: **ptosis**, lid retraction, **proptosis**, chemosis
- **Pupils**: size symmetry, **light response**, RAPD

2) Ocular alignment & movements

- **Cover–uncover** and **alternate cover test** (misalignment)
- **Extraocular movements** (H-pattern) + note pain, limitation, nystagmus
- Localise patterns:
    - **CN VI palsy:** impaired abduction
    - **CN IV palsy:** vertical diplopia worse looking down (stairs), head tilt
    - **CN III palsy:** ptosis, "down and out" ± pupil involvement

3) Neuro exam

- Cranial nerves, cerebellar signs, gait, limb power/sensation
- Fundoscopy if possible: **papilloedema**

C-Core investigations (workup)

Start with: decide likely category

Monocular diplopia (persists with one eye closed)

- Usually ocular: refractive error, dry eye, cataract, corneal irregularity
- **Workup:** slit lamp/ocular exam, refraction; consider urgent ophthalmology if acute painful red eye or sudden visual loss

Binocular diplopia (resolves with either eye closed)

If red flags / acute neuro signs

- **Stroke pathway: CT head ± CT angiography** (or **MRI brain/brainstem** where available/appropriate)
- Suspected aneurysmal 3rd nerve palsy (especially **pupil involved**) → **urgent CTA/MRA** + neurosurgery/neuro
- Suspected cavernous sinus/orbital apex disease → **MRI brain/orbits with contrast** ± MRV; consider ENT/neuro/ophthalmology

If isolated cranial nerve palsy (no other neuro signs)

- **Bloods:** glucose/HbA1c, lipids, BP assessment (microvascular risk)
- **ESR/CRP** if age ≥50 or GCA symptoms (add platelets)
- **Imaging:**
    - Often **urgent imaging** if atypical features: progressive, painful, pupil involvement, age <50, cancer, immunosuppressed
    - If typical microvascular VI palsy (older + vascular RFs) may be monitored with safety-net, but follow local pathway

If myasthenia suspected

- **AChR antibodies** (± MuSK if negative), **ice pack** test (bedside), consider neurophysiology (SFEMG)
- Assess respiratory/bulbar involvement: FVC/NIF if unwell

If thyroid eye disease suspected
- **TSH/FT4**, thyroid antibodies as needed
- **CT/MRI orbits** if significant proptosis, optic neuropathy concern, or atypical

If raised ICP suspected
- **Neuroimaging first** (CT/MRI)
- Then **LP** (opening pressure, CSF) if safe and indicated

Other helpful tests (selected cases)
- **ECG** (AF if TIA/stroke suspicion)
- **Inflammatory/autoimmune** panel only if clinical suspicion (vasculitis, sarcoid, etc.)

Mnemonic for binocular diplopia: VISION

V vascular (e.g. aneurysm, stroke)
I infectious or inflammatory (e.g. meningitis, autoimmune)
S scalp- e.g. giant cell arteritis which affects blood vessels in head)
S sphenoid and skull base trauma.
I increased intracranial pressure (Pseudotumor cerebri)
O onset of new headaches -can signal underlying serious pathology)
N neoplasm-(e.g. a tumor pressing on nerves or blood vessels)

Mnemonic for causes of Monocular diplopia: ABCD

A Astigmatism
B Behavioral: psychogenic
C Cataract, corneal problem
D Dislocated lens

📖 Mnemonic for Red Flag Features in Diplopia: **DANGER**

- **D** – Dilated pupil with CN III palsy → aneurysm (urgent imaging)
- **A** – Acute painful onset → vascular event / carotid-cavernous fistula / giant cell arteritis
- **N** – Neurological signs (hemiparesis, ataxia, dysarthria → brainstem stroke, MS, tumour)
- **G** – Gaze limitation progressive → space-occupying lesion / cavernous sinus pathology
- **E** – Exophthalmos / orbital swelling → thyroid eye disease, orbital cellulitis, tumour
- **R** – Rapid progression or systemic signs → meningitis, encephalitis, malignancy

Dizziness / Vertigo

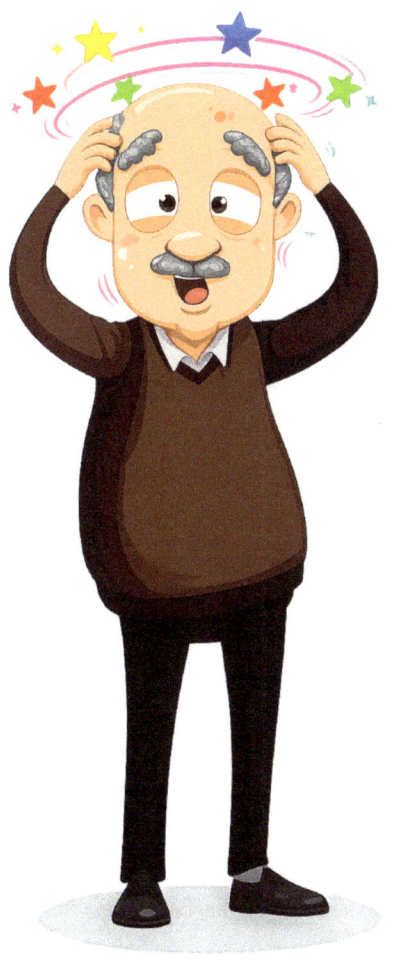

⚑ Red Flags: Dizziness/ Vertigo

- ⚠ Loss of consciousness
- ⚠ Recent Head injury
- ⚠ Acute severe vertigo with new neurological deficits (weakness, dysarthria, diplopia, ataxia, sensory loss)
- ⚠ Sudden onset, prolonged vertigo (hours-days), persistence imbalance
- ⚠ Associated headache, neck pain, or thunderclap headache.
- ⚠ Hearing loss, tinnitus, or aural fullness with vertigo.
- ⚠ Persistent vertigo, progressively worsening imbalance, or new cerebellar signs.
- ⚠ Syncope, collapse, or presyncope associated with dizziness.
- ⚠ Fever, ear pain, or mastoid tenderness with vertigo.
- ⚠ Diplopia, dysarthria, dysphagia, or drop attacks with vertigo.
- ⚠ Elderly with falls, imbalance, or unexplained recurrent vertigo.

∏ **Loss of consciousness:**
- ❖ **Implications/diagnoses:** Postural hypotension, cardiac syncope
- ❖ **Investigations:** L&S BP, ECG/Holter monitor/ Tilt table test and appropriate, ENT referral for vertigo-Dix Hallpike test, Head impulse test.

∏ Recent Head injury:
- ❖ **Implications/Diagnoses:** Traumatic, History of head trauma (e.g., a fall, an assault, or a motor vehicle accident).
- ❖ **Investigations:** Consider CT/ MRI Scan.

∏ Acute severe vertigo with new neurological deficits (weakness, dysarthria, diplopia, ataxia, sensory loss) :
- ❖ **Implications/Diagnoses:** Central lesion (posterior circulation stroke/TIA, brainstem lesion/Tumour, MS).
- ❖ **Investigations:** MRI brain with DWI ± MRA, CT brain (if MRI not available), stroke workup-ECG, Carotid doppler, echocardiogram.

∏ Sudden onset, prolonged vertigo(hours-days), persistence imbalance:
- ❖ **Implications/Diagnoses:** Central cause rather than benign, peripheral- Posterior circulation stroke, vestibular neuritis (if no neuro signs).
- ❖ **Investigations:** MRI brain, HINTS exam (central peripheral), audiogram (to exclude Meniere's).

∏ Associated headache, neck pain , or thunderclap headache:
- ❖ **Implications/Diagnoses:** Vascular pathology or raised ICP- SAH, Vertebral artery dissection, intracranial mass.
- ❖ **Investigations:** CT brain, CTA, LP (if CT negative), MRI brain/spine, MRA (if dissection suspected).

∏ Hearing loss, tinnitus, or aural fullness with vertigo:
- ❖ **Implications/Diagnoses:** Labyrinthine or retrocochlear pathology- Meniere's disease, acoustic neuroma, labyrinthitis.
- ❖ **Investigations:** MRI internal auditory meatus (rule out acoustic neuroma), audiometry (sensorineural hearing loss), Tympanometry/ENT exam.

∏ **Persistent vertigo, progressively worsening imbalance, or new cerebellar signs:**
- **Implications/Diagnoses:** Central lesion (mass, demyelination, degenerative disease)- Cerebellar tumour, MS, degenerative ataxia.
- **Investigations:** MRI brain/posterior fossa, CSF analysis if MS suspected, autoimmune/paraneoplastic panel.

∏ **Syncope, collapse, or presyncope associated with dizziness:**
- **Implications/Diagnoses:** Cardiovascular cause- Arrhythmia, orthostatic hypotension, structural heart disease.
- **Investigations:** ECG, Holter monitor echocardiogram, tilt-table testing, blood-glucose, electrolytes.

∏ **Fever, ear pain, or mastoid tenderness with vertigo:**
- **Implications/Diagnoses:** infectious complication- Otitis media with labyrinthitis, mastoiditis, meningitis.
- **Investigations:** ENT exam, otoscopy, CT temporal bones, MRI brain, FBC, CRP, blood cultures, LP (if meningitis suspected).

∏ **Diplopia, dysphagia, dysarthria or drop attacks with vertigo:**
- **Implications/Diagnoses:** Vertebrobasilar TIA/Stroke.
- **Investigations:** MRI /MRA brain and posterior circulation, CTA vertebral arteries, stroke workup-ECG, bloods.

∏ **Elderly with falls, imbalance, or unexplained recurrent vertigo:**
- **Implications/Diagnoses:** Stroke/TIA, arrhythmia. Neurodegenerative disease.
- **Investigations:** MRI brain, cardiac workup (ECG, Holter, echo), vestibular function tests.

🗝️ Key points:

- Peripheral vertigo- usually benign (BPPV, vestibular neuritis, Meniere's).
- The most common causes of dizziness with vertigo are- BPPV, Meniere's disease, vestibular neuronitis, labyrinthitis.
- Red flags- central signs, neuro deficits, acute severe/persistent vertigo, hearing loss, or systemic illness -urgent imaging and work up.
- MRI brain (posterior fossa) and cardiac tests are important in ruling out life-threatening causes.

ABC approach to Dizziness and vertigo (evaluation + workup):

A — Assessment and immediate threats

1) Rapid severity check

- Obs/NEWS2, SpO_2, HR, BP (include **postural**), temp, **capillary glucose**
- Look for **shock**, arrhythmia, hypoxia, severe dehydration

2) "Can't miss" causes (red flags = urgent same-day / ED / stroke pathway)

- **Posterior circulation stroke/TIA:** acute onset + **focal neurology** (dysarthria, diplopia, ataxia, limb weakness/numbness), inability to walk unaided
- **Cerebellar haemorrhage/infarct:** severe vertigo + headache/vomiting + truncal ataxia
- **Cardiac causes:** chest pain, palpitations, syncope/presyncope, **abnormal ECG**, exertional symptoms
- **Sepsis/meningitis:** fever, rigors, neck stiffness, altered mental state

- **Severe headache** (thunderclap) → SAH pathway
- **GI bleed/anaemia** symptoms: collapse, melena, pallor
- **Toxic/metabolic:** hypoglycaemia, severe electrolyte disturbance

Immediate actions if red flags present
- ABCDE, IV access, fluids if hypotensive/dehydrated
- **ECG**, glucose, treat hypoglycaemia
- **Urgent neuro assessment; CT/MRI** per stroke pathway if central cause suspected

B — Bedside assessment (focused history and exam)

Focused history (aim: vertigo vs presyncope vs imbalance)
- **What do they mean by dizziness?**
  - **Vertigo:** spinning/tilting sensation
  - **Presyncope:** faint/blackout feeling
  - **Disequilibrium:** unsteady gait
- **Timing & triggers (high-yield)**
  - **Seconds, triggered by head movement → BPPV**
  - **Hours with hearing symptoms → Ménière's**
  - **Days, post-viral → vestibular neuritis/labyrinthitis**
  - **Continuous + neuro signs → central (stroke)**
- **Associated symptoms**
  - **Hearing loss/tinnitus/aural fullness** (peripheral)
  - **Headache, diplopia, dysarthria, weakness, numbness** (central)
  - **Chest pain/palpitations** (cardiac)
  - Nausea/vomiting, falls

- **Risk factors**
  - Vascular: HTN, DM, AF, smoking, anticoagulation
  - Migraine history; recent URTI
  - Meds: antihypertensives, diuretics, sedatives, ototoxins; alcohol

Focused exam
- **Vitals + postural BP**
- **Cardio:** pulse rhythm, murmurs, signs of HF
- **Neuro:** cranial nerves, limb power/sensation, cerebellar signs, gait
- **Eye exam (key)**
  - **Nystagmus** (direction-fixed vs direction-changing; vertical = central)
  - **Test of skew** (vertical misalignment suggests central)
- **Bedside vestibular tests**
  - **Dix–Hallpike** if positional vertigo suspected (BPPV)
  - **HINTS** (Head impulse, Nystagmus, Test of skew) **only in continuous acute vestibular syndrome** (vertigo + nystagmus + gait unsteadiness). Central features on HINTS → urgent imaging/stroke pathway.
  - **ENT:** otoscopy (OM, perforation), hearing screen (Weber/Rinne)

C- Core investigations (workup)

Baseline (most patients unless very clear benign BPPV)
- **ECG** (rule out arrhythmia)
- **Capillary glucose**

- **Bloods:** FBC, U&E, CRP (if infection), ± magnesium, thyroid tests if indicated
- Consider **pregnancy test** where relevant

If central cause suspected (red flags, abnormal neuro, central HINTS)

- **Urgent brain imaging** per pathway:
    - Often **MRI brain/brainstem** preferred for posterior circulation
    - CT ± CTA may be initial depending on availability/pathway
- Consider **stroke/TIA workup:** AF screen, carotid/echo if indicated (though posterior often vertebrobasilar)

If peripheral vestibular likely

- **BPPV:** no routine bloods/imaging; treat with **Epley** (after positive Dix–Hallpike)
- **Vestibular neuritis/labyrinthitis:** usually clinical; consider CRP if systemic features; audiology if hearing loss
- **Ménière's:** audiology; ENT referral

If presyncope/orthostatic symptoms

- **Orthostatic vitals**, review meds/volume status
- **FBC** (anaemia), **U&E** (dehydration), consider troponin if chest pain/ACS features
- Consider ambulatory monitoring if intermittent palpitations/syncope features

If infection suspected
- Cultures and imaging targeted to source (e.g., **CXR**, urinalysis) based on symptoms

Mnemonic for Common & Serious Causes of Dizziness/Vertigo: **VESTIBULAR**

- **V** – Vestibular neuritis / Labyrinthitis
- **E** – Ear problems (otitis media, cholesteatoma, Meniere's disease)
- **S** – Stroke (posterior circulation, cerebellar) 🚩
- **T** – Trauma (head injury, perilymph fistula) 🚩
- **I** – Ischaemia (TIA/vertebrobasilar insufficiency) 🚩
- **B** – Benign paroxysmal positional vertigo (BPPV)
- **U** – Unsteady due to drugs (aminoglycosides, anticonvulsants, alcohol), Under hydration (postural hypotension)
- **L** – Lesions/mass(acoustic neuroma, posterior fossa tumour) 🚩
- **A** – Anaemia or arrhythmia 🚩 (systemic causes of presyncope)
- **R** – Reflex/autonomic causes (orthostatic hypotension, vasovagal)

Mnemonic for Red Flags in Dizziness/Vertigo: **BRAIN**

- **B** – Brainstem/cerebellar symptoms: diplopia, dysarthria, dysphagia, limb weakness → stroke/TIA
- **R** – Recent head trauma → intracranial bleed, temporal bone fracture
- **A** – Acute severe continuous vertigo with inability to stand/walk → cerebellar stroke

- **I** – Intractable vomiting / new severe headache → raised ICP, haemorrhage, meningitis
- **N** – New neurological deficits (ataxia, hearing loss, facial weakness, numbness) → posterior fossa lesion

Dyspepsia

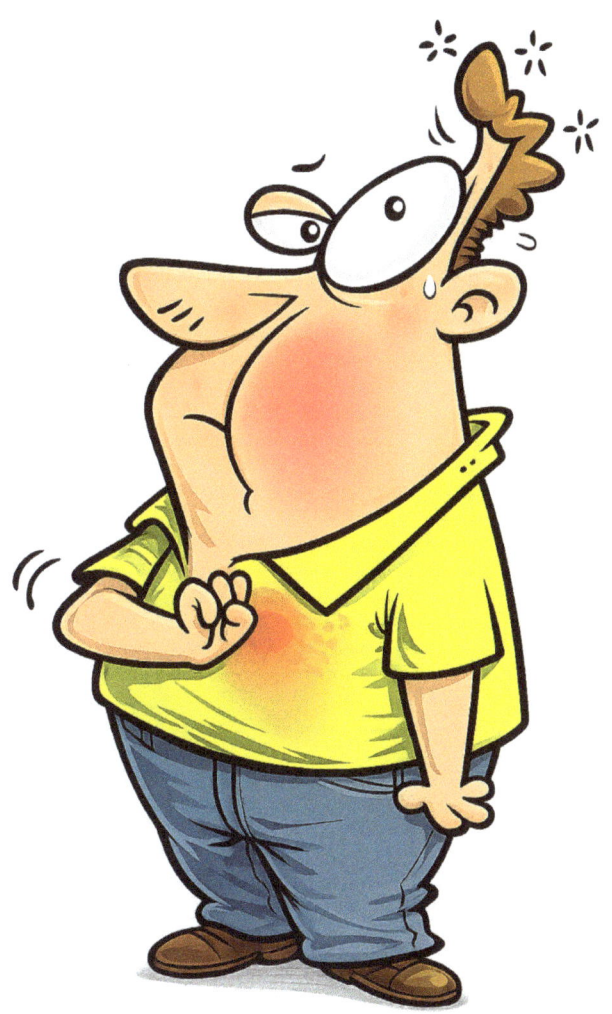

Red Flags: Dyspepsia

- Dysphagia (difficulty swallowing)
- Unintentional weight loss
- Persistent vomiting
- Haematemesis/melaena, blood in stools
- Iron-deficiency anaemia
- Palpable epigastric/abdominal mass
- Age> 55 years with new-onset dyspepsia
- Family history of upper GI cancer or known genetic cancer syndrome
- Progressive dysphagia
- Jaundice
- Persistent or recurrent symptoms despite treatment.

Dysphagia (difficulty swallowing):
- **Implications/Diagnoses:** Oesophageal cancer, strictures, achalasia.
- **Investigations:** OGD(endoscopy).

Unintentional weight loss:
- **Implications/Diagnoses:** Gastric or esophageal malignancy, systemic disease.
- **Investigations:** OGD with biopsy, CT abdomen/pelvis, tumour markers.

Persistent vomiting:
- **Implications/Diagnoses:** Gastric outlet obstruction, malignancy, severe ulcer disease.

- ❖ **Investigations:** OGD, abdominal imaging, (CT, Ultrasound), UEC.

∏ Haematemesis/melaena (GI bleeding):
- ❖ **Implications/Diagnoses:** Peptic ulcer, gastric/esophageal cancer, varices.
- ❖ **Investigations:** OGD, FBC, Coagulation screen, cross-match.

∏ Iron-deficiency anaemia:
- ❖ **Implications/Diagnoses:** Chronic GI blood loss (gastric cancer, peptic ulcer, angiodysplasia).
- ❖ **Investigations:** FBC, Iron studies, OGD + colonoscopy.

∏ Palpable epigastric/abdominal mass:
- ❖ **Implications/Diagnoses:** Gastric malignancy, pancreatic tumour.
- ❖ **Investigations:** OGD, CT TAP, Ultrasound.

∏ Age > 55 years with new-onset dyspepsia:
- ❖ **Implications/Diagnoses:** Malignancy.
- ❖ **Investigations:** OGD with biopsy

∏ Family history of upper GI cancer or known genetic cancer syndrome:
- ❖ **Implications/Diagnoses:** Hereditary cancer risk.
- ❖ **Investigations:** OGD screening/surveillance, genetic counselling.

∏ Progressive dysphagia:
- ❖ **Implications/Diagnoses:** Esophageal cancer, stricture, achalasia.
- ❖ **Investigations:** Endoscopy ± barium swallow.

∏ Jaundice:

- ❖ **Implications/Diagnoses:** Hepatobiliary malignancy, pancreatic cancer.
- ❖ **Investigations:** LFTs, Ultrasound abdomen, CT/MRI pancreas.

∏ Persistent or recurrent symptoms despite treatment:

- ❖ **Implications/Diagnoses:** Functional dyspepsia, H. Pylori infection, malignancy.
- ❖ **Investigations:** H. pylori testing, endoscopy, CT/USS abdomen.

Key points:

- Any red flag in dyspepsia = urgent endoscopy.
- Coronary ischaemia should be suspected for those > 45 or with acute "indigestion".
- Those who don't respond to 4 weeks after PPI therapy should require further workup.

ABC approach to Dyspepsia (evaluation + workup):

A — Assessment and immediate threats

Rapid severity check

- Vitals/NEWS2, pain severity, vomiting, haemodynamic stability.

Immediate threats / red flags (urgent same-day / 2WW as appropriate)

- **Upper GI bleed:** haematemesis, coffee-ground vomit, melaena, syncope, pallor
- **Perforation/acute abdomen:** sudden severe pain, guarding/rigidity, shoulder-tip pain

- **ACS masquerade:** epigastric pain with chest pain, dyspnoea, diaphoresis, risk factors
- **Pancreatitis:** severe epigastric pain radiating to back, persistent vomiting
- **Biliary sepsis/cholangitis:** RUQ pain + fever ± jaundice
- **Oesophageal/gastric cancer red flags: progressive dysphagia, odynophagia, unintentional weight loss**, persistent vomiting, iron-deficiency anaemia, palpable mass
- **Age threshold + new symptoms** (per local pathway), strong FHx upper GI cancer
- **NSAID/anticoagulant risk** with significant symptoms

Immediate actions if red flags

- **ECG + troponin** if any cardiac concern
- **Bloods:** FBC, U&E, LFT, CRP, clotting if bleed suspected
- Resus + urgent endoscopy pathway if bleeding
- Urgent surgical review + CT if perforation suspected

B — Bedside assessment (focused history and exam)

Focused history

- **Symptom character:** epigastric pain/burning, post-prandial fullness, early satiety, bloating, nausea
- **Reflux symptoms:** heartburn, regurgitation, waterbrash
- **Alarm symptoms:** dysphagia, weight loss, persistent vomiting, GI bleeding, anaemia symptoms
- **Triggers:** meals, alcohol, coffee, stress; nocturnal symptoms

- **Medication risks: NSAIDs**, aspirin, steroids, bisphosphonates, iron; anticoagulants
- **H. pylori risk:** prior ulcer, household exposure, high-prevalence country
- **PMH:** PUD, GORD, gallstones, pancreatitis, IHD; smoking
- **Pregnancy** possibility where relevant

Focused exam

- General: pallor, cachexia, dehydration
- Abdomen: epigastric tenderness, RUQ tenderness, guarding/peritonism, masses
- Look for jaundice; check for chest signs if atypical (consider pneumonia) and CVS if cardiac concern

C- Core investigations (workup)

If uncomplicated dyspepsia (no red flags)

- Usually **no routine bloods initially**
- **Test for H. pylori** (per local strategy):
    - **Urea breath test or stool antigen** (preferred)
    - *Avoid testing while on PPI* (can give false negatives—hold PPI ~2 weeks if possible)
- Consider **FBC** if symptoms are persistent or anaemia suspected

If red flags or high-risk features

- **FBC** (anaemia), **U&E**
- **LFTs** if RUQ features/jaundice; **CRP** if infection/inflammation suspected

- **Lipase/amylase** if pancreatitis suspected
- **Urgent endoscopy (OGD)** per pathway (alarm symptoms / concerning features)
- If biliary pathology suspected: **USS RUQ** (± MRCP if cholestatic picture)
- If cardiac concern: **ECG ± troponin**

If symptoms persist despite first-line management
- Ensure adequate trial and adherence (e.g., PPI course)
- Consider:
    - **OGD** (especially if recurrent, refractory, or risk factors)
    - **Coeliac screen** (tTG-IgA + total IgA) if overlapping chronic GI symptoms
    - **Abdominal USS** if RUQ pain or gallstone features

Dyspepsia red flags mnemonic : ALARMS

A Anaemia

L Loss of weight

A Anorexia

R Recent onset of progressive symptoms, Relatives with GI cancer

M Mass, Maelena or hematemesis

S Swallowing difficulty

Mnemonic for Common & Serious Causes of Dyspepsia:
GASTRIC

- **G** – GORD (gastro-oesophageal reflux disease)
- **A** – Alcohol/NSAIDs (drug-induced dyspepsia, gastritis)
- **S** – Stomach ulcer / Peptic ulcer disease (H. pylori)
- **T** – Tumours (gastric cancer, pancreatic cancer, oesophageal cancer) 🚩
- **R** – Reflux oesophagitis / functional dyspepsia
- **I** – Infections (H. pylori, rarely parasites)
- **C** – Cholelithiasis / Biliary disease

Dysphagia

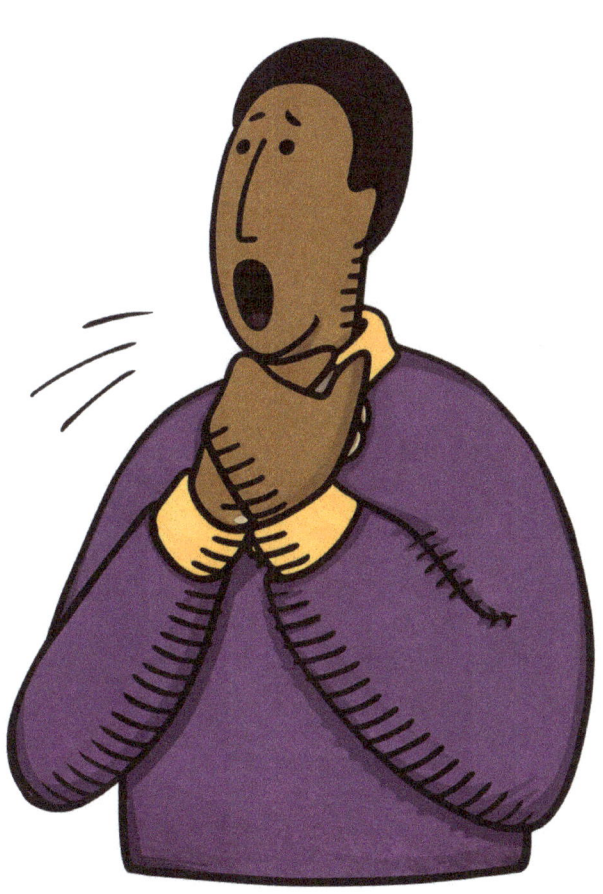

▶ Red Flags: Dysphagia

- ⚠ **Progressive Dysphagia (worsening over weeks to months)**
- ⚠ **Dysphagia to both solids and liquids from onset**
- ⚠ **Rapid weight loss and anorexia**
- ⚠ **Rapid weight loss and anorexia**
- ⚠ **Haematemesis or melaena with dysphagia**
- ⚠ **Associated hoarseness or chronic cough**
- ⚠ **Neurological red flags**
- ⚠ **Odynophagia**
- ⚠ **History of caustic ingestion or radiotherapy**
- ⚠ **Cervical radiotherapy or supraclavicular mass with dysphagia**
- ⚠ **Age > 55 with new onset dysphagia.**

∏ Progressive dysphagia (worsening over weeks to months):
- ❖ **Implications /Diagnoses:** Oesophageal carcinoma, Peptic stricture from GORD.
- ❖ **Investigations:** Urgent upper GI endoscopy (within 2 weeks in suspected cancer, Biopsy, CT chest/abdomen staging if malignancy suspected

∏ Dysphagia to both solids and liquids from onset:
- ❖ **Implications /Diagnoses:** Achalasia, Other motility disorder (e.g., diffuse oesophageal spasm, scleroderma).
- ❖ **Investigations:** Endoscopy (to exclude cancer mimicking motility disorder), Barium swallow (bird-beak in achalasia), Oesophageal manometry (gold standard for motility disorders).

∏ Rapid weight loss and anorexia:
- **Implications /Diagnoses:** Oesophageal or gastric malignancy.
- **Investigations:** upper GI endoscopy with biopsy, CT chest/abdomen for staging.

∏ Haematemesis or melaena with dysphagia:
- **Implications /Diagnoses:** Oesophageal cancer with ulceration, Severe oesophagitis, Varices.
- **Investigations:** Urgent endoscopy with therapeutic capability, coagulation, cross-match.

∏ Associated hoarseness or chronic cough:
- **Implications /Diagnoses:** Laryngeal cancer with invasion, Recurrent laryngeal nerve palsy from mediastinal tumour, Pharyngeal pouch with aspiration.
- **Investigations:** ENT examination + nasoendoscopy, CXR / CT neck and chest, Barium swallow (pharyngeal pouch).

∏ Neurological red flags (sudden onset dysphagia, choking, aspiration, cranial nerve deficits):
- **Implications /Diagnoses:** Acute stroke, Motor neurone disease, Parkinson's, bulbar palsy.
- **Investigations:** Neurological exam, MRI brain (if acute stroke suspected), Video fluoroscopy / swallowing assessment (SALT)

∏ Odynophagia (painful swallowing):
- **Implications/Diagnoses:** Oesophageal cancer with ulceration, Severe oesophagitis (infective in immunosuppressed, e.g., candida, CMV, HSV).
- **Investigations:** Endoscopy with biopsy and cultures.

∏ History of caustic ingestion or previous radiotherapy:
* **Implications /Diagnoses:** Benign stricture, Secondary malignancy
* **Investigations:** Endoscopy with biopsy, Barium swallow if high perforation risk.

∏ Cervical lymphadenopathy or supraclavicular mass with dysphagia:
* **Implications / Diagnoses:** Head and neck malignancy, Metastatic oesophageal/gastric cancer.
* **Investigations:** ENT referral + nasoendoscopy, Neck ultrasound ± FNA, CT neck/chest/abdomen

∏ Age >55 with new onset dysphagia:
* **Implications / Diagnoses:** Oesophageal or gastric cancer until proven otherwise.
* **Investigations:** Urgent endoscopy with biopsy.

🗝 Key points:
* Any patient with dysphagia or >55 years with weight loss + upper GI symptoms → urgent OGD within 2 weeks.
* Solids only → progressive → likely mechanical obstruction (e.g., cancer, stricture).
* Solids + liquids from start → motility disorder (achalasia, spasm).
* Difficulty initiating swallow, nasal regurgitation, aspiration → oropharyngeal / neurological cause.
* Dysphagia is classified as oropharyngeal or Oesophageal.

ABC approach to Dysphagia (evaluation + workup):

A — Assessment and immediate threats

Rapid severity check

- Obs/NEWS2, hydration, ability to swallow **saliva/fluids**, aspiration risk, weight loss, distress.

Immediate threats / red flags (urgent same-day / ED / 2WW as appropriate)

- **Airway compromise / obstruction:** stridor, drooling, inability to swallow saliva, acute distress
- **Food bolus impaction:** sudden dysphagia after eating, chest pain, drooling/retching
- **Aspiration / pneumonia:** cough on swallowing, breathlessness, fever, hypoxia
- **Stroke/brainstem signs:** acute onset dysphagia + dysarthria, facial droop, limb weakness, ataxia
- **Oesophageal perforation:** severe chest pain after vomiting/instrumentation, subcutaneous emphysema, sepsis
- **Cancer red flags: progressive dysphagia (solids → liquids)**, **weight loss**, persistent vomiting, **iron-deficiency anaemia**, odynophagia, palpable neck nodes
- **Caustic ingestion** or severe pill injury (bisphosphonates, doxycycline)

Immediate actions

- **NBM** if aspiration risk/unsafe swallow; sit upright
- If food bolus: urgent **endoscopy pathway** (and airway protection if needed)

- If stroke suspected: **stroke pathway** + urgent imaging
- Treat sepsis/aspiration pneumonia as indicated; early speech & language therapy (SALT) involvement

B — Bedside assessment (focused history and exam)

Focused history (localise: oropharyngeal vs Oesophageal)

Key discriminator

- **Oropharyngeal dysphagia:** difficulty *initiating* swallow, choking/coughing, nasal regurgitation, "wet" voice
- Red Flags
- **Oesophageal dysphagia:** food "sticks" after swallowing, retrosternal discomfort

Character & pattern

- **Solids only** (structural obstruction/stricture/cancer) vs **solids + liquids** (motility disorder)
- **Intermittent** (rings/webs/spasm) vs **progressive** (malignancy/stricture)
- **Odynophagia** (inflammation: oesophagitis, candida, pill injury)
- Reflux symptoms, long-standing heartburn (peptic stricture/Barrett's risk)
- Neurology symptoms (stroke, Parkinson's, MND, MS), weight loss, night sweats
- Aspiration symptoms: recurrent chest infections, coughing with meals
- Meds: anticholinergics (dry mouth), opioids, bisphosphonates, doxycycline, NSAIDs

- Risk factors: smoking, alcohol, head/neck cancer, immunosuppression

Focused exam

- General: hydration, cachexia, fever, voice quality ("wet voice"), drooling
- Mouth/throat: oral candidiasis, dental status, tonsillar/pharyngeal lesions
- Neuro: cranial nerves (IX, X, XII), gag (limited value), bulbar signs
- Chest: aspiration signs
- Neck: lymphadenopathy, masses

C-Core investigations (workup)

First-line based on risk

- **Urgent OGD** if:
  - Progressive dysphagia, weight loss, anaemia, GI bleeding, odynophagia, persistent vomiting
  - Suspected food bolus/obstruction (emergency)
- **CXR** if aspiration suspected; consider ABG/VBG if hypoxic

Oropharyngeal dysphagia suspected

- **Bedside swallow screen** (stroke pathway) + **SALT assessment**
- **Videofluoroscopy (modified barium swallow)** or **FEES** (fibreoptic endoscopic evaluation of swallow)
- Consider **MRI/CT brain** if new neuro deficits or unclear cause

Oesophageal dysphagia suspected
- **OGD** (diagnostic ± biopsy; can dilate strictures)
- **Barium swallow if:**
  - Suspected high oesophageal/ pharyngeal pouch, rings/webs, or if OGD not possible/initially non-diagnostic
- **Oesophageal manometry** if OGD normal and motility disorder suspected (achalasia, spasm)
- **pH/impedance testing** if reflux-related symptoms persist despite therapy and diagnosis uncertain

Baseline labs (often useful)
- **FBC** (anaemia), **U&E** (dehydration), **CRP** if infection/inflammation suspected
- Consider LFTs, albumin if weight loss/malnutrition

Mnemonic for causes of Dysphagia: **DYS-PHAGIA**

D **Diverticula** (e.g. pharyngeal pouch-regurgitation, aspiration.

Y **Young -Neurological** (stroke, MND, PD, MS, bulbar palsy) 🚩

S **Stricture** (benign peptic stricture, caustic ingestion, radiotherapy)

P **Pharyngeal causes** (globus, achalasia,)

H **Head/neck cancer** (oropharyngeal, laryngeal, oesophageal) 🚩

A **Achalasia / motility disorders** (achalasia, scleroderma, oesophageal spasm)

G **Gastro-oesophageal reflux** (commonest; leading to oesophagitis, peptic stricture, Barrett's)

I **Infections / Inflammation** (candida, HSV, CMV, eosinophilic oesophagitis)

A **Anatomical anomalies** (webs, rings – e.g., Schatzki's ring, Plummer–Vinson)

Mnemonic for Red Flags in Dysphagia: CHOKE

- **C – Cancer clues** → progressive dysphagia, especially solids → liquids
- **H – Haematemesis / anaemia** (GI bleeding, iron deficiency)
- **O – Older age / Onset recent** (>55 years, new or rapidly progressive)
- **K – Kilogram loss** (unexplained weight loss, anorexia)
- **E – Extra symptoms** → aspiration, recurrent pneumonia, voice change, neck mass, odynophagia (painful swallowing)

Dyspnoea

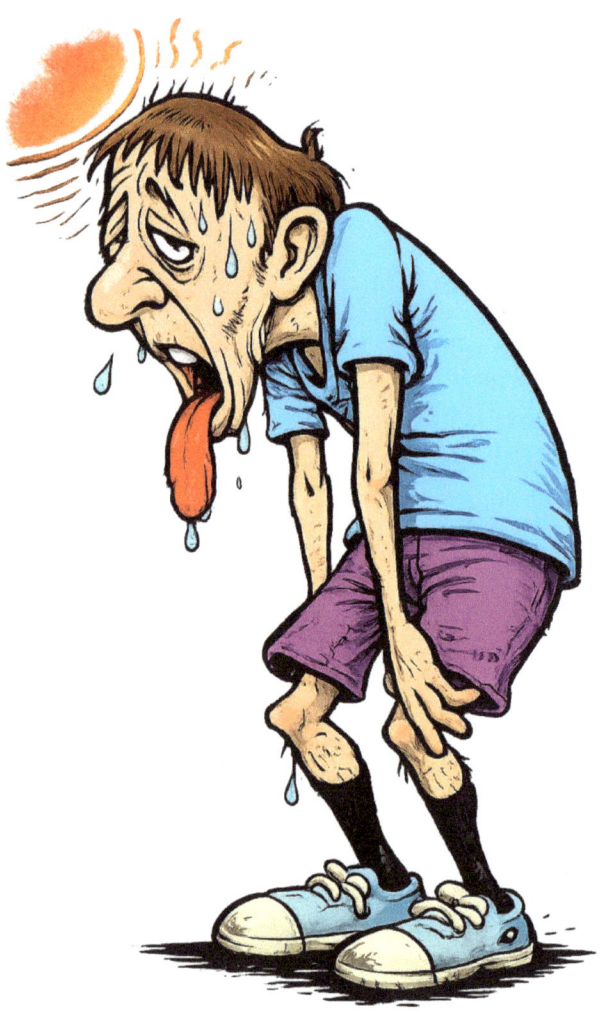

▶ Red Flags: Dyspnoea

- ⚠ Acute severe breathlessness, sudden onset:
- ⚠ Breathlessness with chest pain (pleuritic or central)
- ⚠ Haemoptysis (coughing blood)
- ⚠ Stridor, noisy breathing, inability to complete sentences:
- ⚠ Severe hypoxia (SpO_2 < 90% on air)
- ⚠ Orthopnoea, paroxysmal nocturnal dyspnoea, pink frothy sputum
- ⚠ Weight loss, night sweats, chronic cough:
- ⚠ Fever, rigors, purulent sputum, confusion (esp. elderly)
- ⚠ Dyspnoea after immobilisation, surgery, or long travel with pleuritic pain and tachycardia
- ⚠ Dyspnoea with calf swelling/pain and raised JVP
- ⚠ Sudden collapse, hypotension or shock with dyspnoea
- ⚠ Progressive exertional dyspnoea with clubbing or cyanosis
- ⚠ Chronic cough, smoking history with worsening breathlessness
- ⚠ Haemodynamic instability (tachycardia, hypotension, syncope with breathlessness)
- ⚠ Widespread wheeze or crackles

∏ Acute severe breathlessness, sudden onset:
- ❖ **Implications/Diagnoses**, pneumothorax, acute asthma/COPD exacerbation.

- ❖ **Investigations:** Chest X-ray, ECG, ABG, D-dimer ± CTPA, CT chest, peak flow/spirometry.

∏ Breathlessness with chest pain (pleuritic or central):
- ❖ **Implications/Diagnoses:** PE, acute coronary syndrome/MI, pneumothorax, pneumonia.
- ❖ **Investigations:** ECG, troponin, CXR, ABG, CTPA, echocardiography if needed.

∏ Haemoptysis (coughing blood):
- ❖ **Implications/Diagnoses:** Lung cancer, massive PE, tuberculosis, bronchiectasis, severe pneumonia.
- ❖ **Investigations:** Urgent CXR, CT chest, sputum culture/AFB, bronchoscopy.

∏ Stridor, noisy breathing, inability to complete sentences:
- ❖ **Implications/Diagnoses:** Upper airway obstruction, anaphylaxis, severe asthma.
- ❖ **Investigations:** ABG, nasoendoscopy/bronchoscopy, urgent ENT/anaesthetic review.

∏ Severe hypoxia (SpO_2 < 90% on air):
- ❖ **Implications/Diagnoses:** Respiratory failure (Type 1 or 2) due to pneumonia, PE, ARDS, acute asthma/COPD.
- ❖ **Investigations:** ABG, CXR, ECG, bloods (FBC, U&E, CRP, troponin).

∏ Orthopnoea, paroxysmal nocturnal dyspnoea, pink frothy sputum:
- ❖ **Implications/Diagnoses:** Acute left ventricular failure / pulmonary oedema.
- ❖ **Investigations:** CXR, BNP/NT-proBNP, ECG, echo, ABG.

⨿ Weight loss, night sweats, chronic cough:

- **Implications/Diagnoses:** Lung cancer, tuberculosis, interstitial lung disease.
- **Investigations:** CXR, CT chest, sputum AFB/culture, PET scan, biopsy.

⨿ Fever, rigors, purulent sputum, confusion (esp. elderly):

- **Implications/Diagnoses:** Severe pneumonia, sepsis.
- **Investigations:** CXR, FBC, CRP, blood cultures, ABG, CURB-65 severity scoring.

⨿ Dyspnoea after immobilisation, surgery, or long travel with pleuritic pain and tachycardia:

- **Implications/Diagnoses:** Pulmonary embolism.
- **Investigations:** Wells score, D-dimer, CTPA, ECG, troponin.

⨿ Dyspnoea with calf swelling/pain and raised JVP:

- **Implications/Diagnoses:** PE, right heart strain.
- **Investigations:** CTPA, Doppler leg ultrasound, ECG, troponin, echo.

⨿ Sudden collapse, hypotension or shock with dyspnoea:

- **Implications/Diagnoses:** Massive PE, tension pneumothorax, myocardial infarction, cardiac tamponade, septic shock.
- **Investigations:** Bedside echo/ultrasound, ECG, CXR, ABG, urgent CT chest.

⨿ Progressive exertional dyspnoea with clubbing or cyanosis:

- **Implications/Diagnoses:** Interstitial lung disease, pulmonary fibrosis, lung cancer.
- **Investigations:** CXR, high-resolution CT, spirometry, 6-minute walk test, lung biopsy.

∏ **Chronic cough, smoking history with worsening breathlessness:**
- ❖ **Implications/Diagnoses:** COPD exacerbation, lung cancer.
- ❖ **Investigations:** CXR, spirometry, ABG, CT chest.

∏ **Haemodynamic instability (tachycardia, hypotension, syncope with breathlessness):**
- ❖ **Implications/Diagnoses:** Massive PE, tamponade, acute MI, severe sepsis.
- ❖ **Investigations:** ECG, echo, CXR, troponin, ABG, CT chest, blood cultures.

∏ **Widespread wheeze or crackles:**
- ❖ **Implications/Diagnoses:** Asthma, COPD, LVF
- ❖ **Investigations:** Chest X-ray : Upper lobe diversion, Kerley B Lines - indicate pulmonary edema, hyperinflated lung in COPD.

🗝 Key Points:

- The most common causes overall are- Pneumonia, asthma, COPD, heart failure/myocardial ischaemia and deconditioning.
- Low Oxygen saturations (<90%) is indicative of a significant underlying problem but normal saturations does not rule out.
- Accessory muscle use, low oxygen saturations, high respiratory rate or decreased level of consciousness require urgent and immediate evaluation.
- Known chronic conditions (e.g heart failure, asthma, COPD) can present with exacerbations commonly but such patients can also
- The most common ca

ABC approach to Dyspnoea (evaluation + workup):

A — Assessment and immediate threats

Rapid severity check (ABCDE)

- Obs/NEWS2: **SpO$_2$**, RR, HR, BP, temp, conscious level; look for **fatigue/exhaustion**.
- Start **oxygen if hypoxic**, sit upright, nebulisers if wheeze, IV access if unwell.

Immediate threats / red flags (treat now + urgent pathway)

- **Airway obstruction/anaphylaxis:** stridor, wheeze + hypotension, urticaria, angioedema → IM adrenaline, airway help
- **Life-threatening asthma/COPD:** silent chest, exhaustion, rising CO_2 → nebs, steroids, ABG, consider NIV/ITU
- **Pulmonary embolism:** pleuritic pain, tachycardia, hypoxia, syncope, DVT signs → PE pathway (D-dimer/CTPA)
- **Pneumothorax:** sudden pleuritic pain + unilateral reduced breath sounds; tension signs (hypotension, tracheal shift) → immediate decompression
- **Acute pulmonary oedema/HF:** orthopnoea, crackles, pink froth → nitrates/diuretics/NIV as indicated
- **ACS/arrhythmia:** chest pain, diaphoresis, palpitations, syncope → ECG, troponin, manage per pathway
- **Sepsis/pneumonia:** fever, hypotension, confusion → sepsis bundle + antibiotics

- **Metabolic acidosis:** Kussmaul breathing, DKA/renal failure/toxins → VBG/ABG + targeted treatment

B — Bedside assessment (focused history and exam)

Focused history

- **Onset:** sudden vs gradual; duration; progression; episodic vs constant
- **Triggers:** exertion, lying flat, allergens, infection, travel/immobility
- **Associated symptoms:**
    - **Chest pain** (pleuritic vs central), cough/sputum, haemoptysis
    - Wheeze, fever, leg swelling/pain, palpitations/syncope
    - Orthopnoea/PND, weight gain (HF), anxiety symptoms (after ruling out organic causes)
- **Past history:** asthma/COPD, HF/IHD, VTE, malignancy, ILD, anaemia, renal disease
- **Risk factors:** smoking, OCP/pregnancy, recent surgery, immobilisation, AF
- **Medication:** beta-blockers, sedatives/opioids, recent changes; anticoagulation status

Focused exam

- **General:** ability to speak, accessory muscle use, cyanosis, sweating
- **Chest:** wheeze (asthma/COPD), crackles (HF/pneumonia/ILD), unilateral changes (pneumothorax/effusion)
- **CVS:** JVP, oedema, murmurs, irregular pulse

- **Peripheral:** calf swelling/tenderness (DVT), pallor (anaemia)
- **Bedside:** peak flow (known asthma), capillary glucose if unwell

C- Core investigations (workup)

Core tests for most acute dyspnoea

- **Pulse oximetry ± ABG/VBG** (if hypoxic, severe COPD/asthma, drowsy, or shock)
- **ECG**
- **CXR**
- **Bloods: FBC, U&E, CRP** ± LFT
- **Troponin** if chest pain/ACS concern
- **BNP/NT-proBNP** if HF suspected

Targeted tests (based on likely cause)

- **PE:** D-dimer (if low/intermediate risk) → **CTPA** if indicated (or V/Q if appropriate)
- **Infection:** blood cultures if septic; sputum culture if productive; viral testing in season
- **Asthma/COPD:** peak flow; later **spirometry** when stable
- **Pneumothorax/effusion:** bedside **lung ultrasound** if available; CXR confirmation; CT if uncertain
- **Anaemia/bleed:** FBC trend; iron studies if chronic
- **Metabolic:** glucose/ketones, lactate, bicarbonate; consider DKA/toxin screen if suggested
- **Chronic/unexplained:** CT chest, echo, PFTs, sleep study, depending on pattern

📋 Mnemonic for Common & Serious Causes of Dyspnoea: "HEART LUNG"

👉 **Covers common + serious causes**

H – Heart failure → LV failure, pulmonary oedema, cardiomyopathy

E – Embolism → Pulmonary embolism

A – Asthma / COPD exacerbation → Bronchospasm, airway limitation

R – Respiratory infection → Pneumonia, bronchitis, COVID, sepsis

T – Tension pneumothorax → Sudden dyspnoea, chest pain, collapse

L – Lung cancer / mass → Obstructive or malignant cause

U – Upper airway obstruction / anaphylaxis → Stridor, swelling

N – Neuromuscular weakness → Myasthenia, Guillain–Barré, MND

G – Gas exchange / metabolic → Anaemia, acidosis, obesity hypoventilation

✅ **Tip:** "HEART LUNG" = think both **cardiac and respiratory** causes that kill.

📋 Mnemonic for Red Flags in Dyspnoea: "BREATHLESS"

B – Blue lips / severe hypoxia (SpO$_2$ < 90%) → Respiratory failure

R – Rapid onset / sudden collapse → PE, pneumothorax, MI

E – Exhaustion / inability to talk in sentences → Severe asthma/COPD

A – Accessory muscle use / stridor → Airway obstruction, anaphylaxis

T – Tachycardia / hypotension / shock → Massive PE, sepsis, tamponade

H – Haemoptysis → Lung cancer, TB, PE

L – Left heart failure signs (PND, orthopnoea, frothy sputum) → Pulmonary oedema

E – Elderly with confusion + fever → Severe pneumonia, sepsis

S – Smoker with weight loss / persistent cough → Lung cancer

S – Sudden postoperative / post-flight dyspnoea → PE

Dysuria

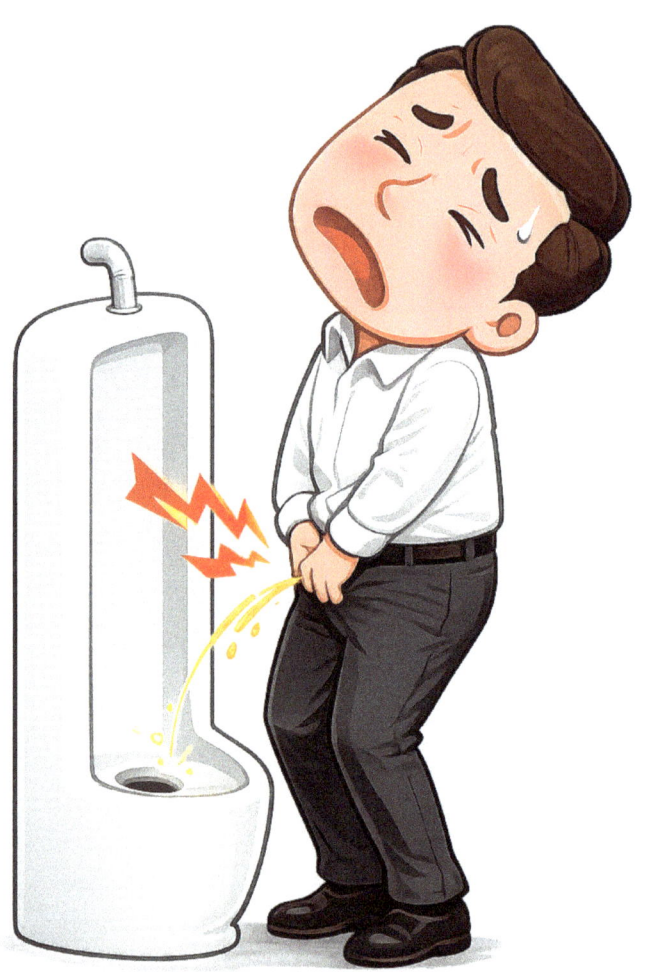

Red Flags: Dysuria

- ⚠ Fever, rigors, flank pain or costovertebral angle tenderness
- ⚠ Visible (macroscopic) haematuria:
- ⚠ Recurrent or persistent dysuria not responding to treatment
- ⚠ Haematuria with clots or passage of tissue:
- ⚠ Dysuria with urinary retention or poor stream (especially in men)
- ⚠ Dysuria with genital ulcers, discharge, or perineal pain
- ⚠ Systemic unwellness – hypotension, tachycardia, confusion (especially in elderly)
- ⚠ Suprapubic pain with retention or acute abdominal signs
- ⚠ Pain in the flank, groin, or radiating to the testicle / labia
- ⚠ Dysuria with new-onset incontinence or neurological symptoms
- ⚠ Immunocompromised patient, Known urinary tract abnormality

∏ Fever, rigors, flank pain or costovertebral angle tenderness:
- ❖ **Implications / Diagnoses:** Pyelonephritis, Urosepsis.
- ❖ **Investigations:** Urinalysis & urine culture, FBC, CRP, U&E, Blood cultures, Renal ultrasound or CT KUB (if obstruction suspected).

∏ Visible (macroscopic) haematuria:
- **Implications / Diagnoses:** Bladder or renal malignancy, Renal stones, Glomerulonephritis.
- **Investigations:** Urinalysis for blood and protein, Urine cytology, Ultrasound KUB ± CT urogram, Cystoscopy, FBC, U&E, eGFR.

∏ Recurrent or persistent dysuria not responding to treatment:
- **Implications / Diagnoses:** Chronic prostatitis (men), Bladder cancer or carcinoma in situ, Interstitial cystitis, Drug-induced or radiation cystitis.
- **Investigations:** Midstream urine (MSU), Cystoscopy ± biopsy, Urine cytology, STI screen (chlamydia, gonorrhoea, mycoplasma).

∏ Haematuria with clots or passage of tissue:
- **Implications / Diagnoses:** Bladder or renal tumour, Renal papillary necrosis, Trauma.
- **Investigations:** Urine microscopy, Imaging (CT urogram / renal ultrasound), Cystoscopy, FBC, U&E, coagulation profile.

∏ Dysuria with urinary retention or poor stream (especially in men):
- **Implications / Diagnoses:** Prostatic enlargement or carcinoma, Urethral stricture, Neurogenic bladder.
- **Investigations:** Post-void bladder scan / residual volume, PSA (if appropriate), Renal function, urinalysis, Ultrasound KUB ± cystoscopy.

∏ Dysuria with genital ulcers, discharge, or perineal pain:
- **Implications / Diagnoses:** Sexually transmitted infections (gonorrhoea, chlamydia, HSV, trichomonas), Prostatitis (men)

- ❖ **Investigations:** Urine NAAT for chlamydia/gonorrhoea, Genital swabs and culture, HIV, syphilis, HSV serology, MSU for culture.

⛳ Systemic unwellness – hypotension, tachycardia, confusion (especially in elderly):

- ❖ **Implications / Diagnoses:** Urosepsis.
- ❖ **Investigations:** Sepsis screen: blood cultures, FBC, CRP, lactate, Urine culture, Renal profile, Imaging if obstruction suspected (CT KUB, ultrasound).

⛳ Suprapubic pain with retention or acute abdominal signs:

- ❖ **Implications / Diagnoses:** Acute urinary retention, Bladder rupture (trauma, instrumentation), Severe cystitis with obstruction
- ❖ **Investigations:** Bladder scan for retention, Catheterisation with measurement of residual volume, CT cystogram (if rupture suspected).

⛳ Pain in the flank, groin, or radiating to the testicle / labia:

- ❖ **Implications / Diagnoses:** Ureteric stones, Pyelonephritis
- ❖ **Investigations:** Urinalysis (haematuria, nitrites), Non-contrast CT KUB, FBC, U&E, CRP, Urine culture.

⛳ Dysuria with new-onset incontinence or neurological symptoms:

- ❖ **Implications / Diagnoses:** Spinal cord compression or cauda equina syndrome, Neurogenic bladder.
- ❖ **Investigations:** Neurological examination, MRI spine (if red flag features), Post-void residual scan, Urinalysis, U&E.

⛳ Immunocompromised patient:

- ❖ **Implications/Diagnoses:** Infections, Sepsis.
- ❖ **Investigations:** Sepsis screen, bloods, CT/USS imaging.

🗝️ Key Points:

- Dysuria is not always caused by bladder infection.
- Most common causes are Cystitis and urethritis from STD.

ABC approach to Dysuria (evaluation + workup):

A — Assessment and immediate threats

Rapid severity check

- Obs/NEWS2, pain score, hydration, ability to pass urine, sepsis screen.

Immediate threats / red flags (urgent same-day / ED)

- **Sepsis / pyelonephritis:** fever/rigors, flank pain, vomiting, hypotension, confusion
- **Obstructed infected system:** dysuria/UTI symptoms + **loin pain + anuria/AKI** or known stone → urgent urology
- **Acute urinary retention:** inability to void, suprapubic pain/distension
- **Testicular torsion/epididymo-orchitis red flags (men):** acute severe scrotal pain/swelling
- **Pregnancy + UTI symptoms** (higher risk complications)
- **Immunosuppressed** / renal transplant / severe comorbidity
- **Visible haematuria** or clots
- **Severe pelvic pain** or peritonism (consider non-urinary causes)

Immediate actions if red flags

- IV access ± fluids, analgesia/antiemetic
- **Urine dip + culture** ASAP (before antibiotics if possible)
- **Bloods:** FBC, U&E/creatinine, CRP ± lactate/blood cultures if septic
- **Pregnancy test** where relevant
- Consider **urgent imaging** (CT KUB/renal USS) if obstruction/stone suspected
- Catheterise if retention (per local policy) + consider urology review

B — Bedside assessment (focused history and exam)

Focused history

- **Symptoms:** burning/pain on urination, frequency, urgency, suprapubic pain
- **Upper tract features: flank pain**, fever, rigors, nausea/vomiting
- **Haematuria:** visible vs microscopic, clots
- **Vaginal symptoms (women):** discharge/itching (vaginitis), dyspareunia
- **Sexual history / STI risk:** new partner, urethral discharge, genital ulcers
- **Urinary flow/obstruction:** weak stream, hesitancy, incomplete emptying (BPH)
- **Stone features:** colicky loin-to-groin pain
- **Recent instrumentation/catheter**, recent antibiotics
- **Pregnancy**, diabetes, immunosuppression, past UTIs

Focused exam

- Vitals, hydration
- **Abdominal:** suprapubic tenderness/distension (retention)
- **CVA tenderness** (pyelonephritis)
- **External genital exam** if discharge/lesions/pain suggests STI/vaginitis (as appropriate)
- **DRE** in men if prostatitis/BPH suspected (avoid vigorous prostate massage)

C- Core investigations (workup)

Initial tests (most cases)

- **Urine dipstick** (nitrites, leukocytes, blood)
- **Urine culture (MSU) if:** male, pregnant, recurrent/complicated UTI, pyelonephritis, immunosuppressed, catheter-associated, treatment failure
- **Pregnancy test** in women of childbearing potential

Blood tests (if systemically unwell or complicated)

- **FBC, U&E/creatinine, CRP**
- **Blood cultures** ± lactate if septic

STI/vaginal cause suspected

- **NAAT** for chlamydia/gonorrhoea (first-void urine or swab per pathway)
- Vaginal swabs/pH microscopy depending on services (BV/candida/trichomonas)

Imaging (when indicated)

- **Renal ultrasound if:** suspected obstruction, recurrent UTIs, pregnancy with flank pain, AKI, known stones/hydronephrosis risk

- **CT KUB** if stone suspected (non-pregnant) or diagnosis unclear
- Consider urology referral for **visible haematuria** or persistent microscopic haematuria per local pathway

Mnemonic for Common & Serious Causes of Dysuria: "PAINFUL"

👉 Each letter stands for a key *common or serious* cause of dysuria

P – Pyelonephritis / Prostatitis
Upper UTI or prostate infection causing flank or perineal pain.

A – Acute cystitis (UTI)
Most common cause, bacterial infection (E. coli, etc.).

I – Infections (STIs)
Chlamydia, Gonorrhoea, Trichomonas, HSV, Mycoplasma.

N – Nephrolithiasis (renal / ureteric stones)
Dysuria with flank pain or haematuria.

F – Foreign body / catheter irritation / trauma
Instrumentation, catheter, or sexual trauma.

U – Urethritis / Urinary obstruction
From STI, BPH, stricture, or malignancy.

L – Lesions / malignancy of bladder or urethra
Bladder carcinoma, carcinoma in situ, or ulceration.

✅ *Tip:* "PAINFUL" = the **PAINFUL** causes of dysuria.

📖 Mnemonic for Red Flags in Dysuria: **"BLOODY URINE"**

👉 Each letter represents a **red flag feature** needing urgent attention:

B – Blood in urine (visible haematuria) → Bladder or renal cancer, stones.

L – Loin pain or flank tenderness → Pyelonephritis, obstruction, stones.

O – Old age with new-onset dysuria or haematuria → Malignancy until proven otherwise.

O – Oliguria or urinary retention → Obstruction, prostate enlargement, renal failure.

D – Dysuria with fever, rigors, systemic unwellness → Pyelonephritis, urosepsis.

Y – Young man with perineal pain / poor stream → Acute prostatitis.

U – Unresolved or recurrent symptoms despite antibiotics → Bladder tumour, resistant infection.

R – Reduced GFR / raised creatinine → Obstruction or sepsis-related AKI.

I – Immunocompromised / diabetic with dysuria → Complicated UTI or fungal infection.

N – Neurological symptoms or incontinence → Cauda equina, neurogenic bladder.

E – Elderly confusion or sepsis picture → Urosepsis.

✅ *Tip:* "BLOODY URINE" = if your patient's urine is **bloody or they look unwell**, think **red flag** — act fast, investigate, and escalate.

Edema

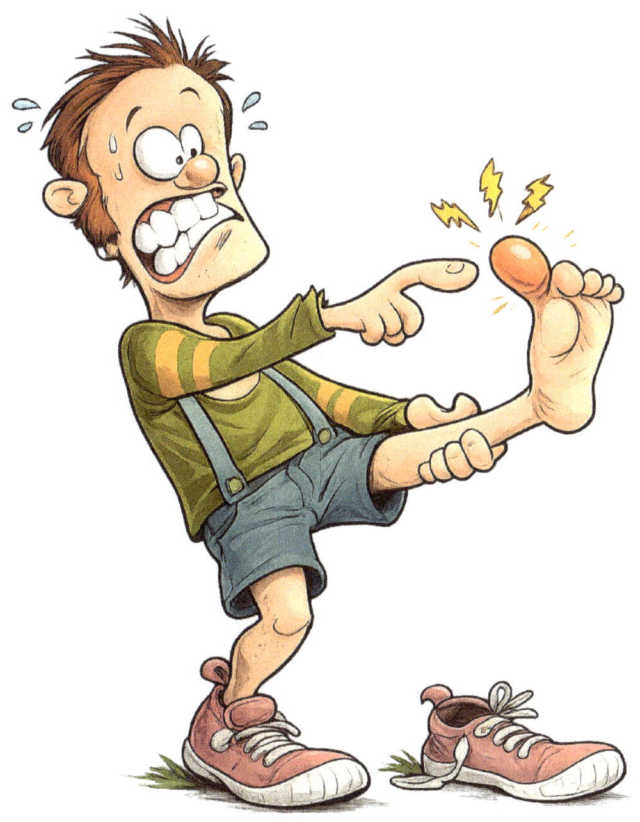

▶ Red Flags: Edema

- ⚠ **Rapid onset oedema (hours to days)**
- ⚠ **Unilateral painful swelling**
- ⚠ **Generalised oedema with dyspnoea or orthopnoea**
- ⚠ **Oedema associated with oliguria or frothy urine**
- ⚠ **Facial or periorbital oedema (especially morning)**
- ⚠ **Oedema with jaundice, ascites, spider naevi**
- ⚠ **Oedema with pleural effusion or raised JVP**
- ⚠ **Oedema with weight loss, fatigue, lymphadenopathy**
- ⚠ **Oedema with hypotension, tachycardia or rash**
- ⚠ **Oedema in pregnancy (especially sudden facial/hand swelling, headache, visual changes)**

∏ Rapid onset oedema (hours to days):
- ❖ **Implications / Diagnoses:** Acute heart failure (left or right), Acute renal failure / nephrotic syndrome, Deep vein thrombosis (DVT), Allergic reaction / angioedema.
- ❖ **Key Investigations:** ECG, BNP, echocardiogram, Serum creatinine, urea, electrolytes, urinalysis, Doppler ultrasound (DVT), CXR (pulmonary oedema), Allergy screen if appropriate.

∏ Unilateral painful swelling:
- ❖ **Implications / Diagnoses:** DVT – most common red flag for unilateral oedema, Cellulitis (warm, erythematous, tender), Lymphatic obstruction / malignancy.
- ❖ **Key Investigations:** D-dimer, duplex Doppler venous ultrasound, CRP (infection), CT / MRI venogram or

lymphoscintigraphy (if malignancy or lymphatic obstruction suspected).

∏ Generalised oedema with dyspnoea or orthopnoea:
- **Implications / Diagnoses:** Congestive cardiac failure, Nephrotic syndrome, Hepatic cirrhosis / portal hypertension.
- **Key Investigations:** BNP, echocardiography, ECG (cardiac),LFTs, albumin, coagulation profile (hepatic),Urinalysis for protein, U&E.

∏ Oedema associated with oliguria or frothy urine:
- **Implications / Diagnoses:** Renal disease / nephrotic syndrome / glomerulonephritis,
- **Key Investigations:** Urinalysis (protein, blood, casts), Serum creatinine, eGFR, U&E, Renal ultrasound, Autoimmune screen (ANA, ANCA, complements).

∏ Facial or periorbital oedema (especially morning):
- **Implications / Diagnoses:** Nephrotic syndrome / glomerulonephritis, Angioedema / allergic reaction,
- **Key Investigations:** Urinalysis (proteinuria, haematuria), U&E, creatinine, Complement levels (C3, C4), immunology, Consider allergy testing (C1 esterase inhibitor levels).

∏ Oedema with jaundice, ascites, spider naevi:
- **Implications / Diagnoses:** Liver failure / cirrhosis / portal hypertension.
- **Key Investigations:** LFTs, albumin, bilirubin, INR, Ultrasound abdomen (liver size, ascites), Hepatitis serology, autoimmune screen.

∏ Oedema with pleural effusion or raised JVP:
- **Implications / Diagnoses:** Right heart failure / constrictive pericarditis / pulmonary hypertension.

- ❖ **Key Investigations:** Echocardiogram, ECG, BNP, CXR, CT chest if pulmonary hypertension suspected.

∏ Oedema with weight loss, fatigue, lymphadenopathy:
- ❖ **Implications / Diagnoses:** Malignancy (lymphoma, metastatic cancer-causing lymphatic obstruction or SVC syndrome).
- ❖ **Key Investigations:** CT chest/abdomen/pelvis, Tumour markers if relevant, ESR, CRP, Biopsy of any palpable lymph nodes.

∏ Oedema with hypotension, tachycardia or rash:
- ❖ **Implications / Diagnoses:** Anaphylaxis or sepsis.
- ❖ **Key Investigations:** Serum tryptase (for anaphylaxis), Blood cultures, inflammatory markers (for sepsis).

∏ Oedema in pregnancy (especially sudden facial/hand swelling, headache, visual changes):
- ❖ **Implications / Diagnoses:** Pre-eclampsia or HELLP syndrome.
- ❖ **Key Investigations:** BP measurement, urinalysis for protein, U&E, LFTs, platelets, Foetal assessment (ultrasound, Doppler).

🔑 Key points:
- ❖ Generalised edema is most commonly caused by- heart failure, Liver failure, Kidney disorders (nephrotic syndrome).
- ❖ Localised edema is most commonly caused by- DVT or another venous obstruction (e.g. by tumour), infection, angioedema, lymphatic obstruction.
- ❖ In the elderly look for drugs causing edema.
- ❖ Sudden onset should trigger prompt evaluation.

ABC approach to edema (evaluation + workup)

A — Assessment and immediate threats

Rapid severity check

- Obs/NEWS2, **SpO$_2$**, RR, HR, BP; assess rapid progression, pain, erythema, dyspnoea.

Immediate threats / red flags (urgent same-day / ED)

- **Anaphylaxis / angioedema** (facial/tongue swelling, stridor, wheeze, hypotension) → airway + IM adrenaline
- **Pulmonary oedema / acute HF** (acute breathlessness, orthopnoea, crackles, hypoxia) → oxygen/NIV, diuretics per pathway
- **DVT / PE** (unilateral painful swollen leg ± dyspnoea/pleuritic pain) → VTE pathway (D-dimer/US Doppler/CTPA)
- **Cellulitis / necrotising infection** (hot, red, very tender, systemic toxicity) → urgent antibiotics/surgical review if nec fasc concern
- **Acute renal failure / severe fluid overload** (oliguria, rising creatinine, hyperkalaemia, pulmonary symptoms) → urgent bloods, ECG, renal review
- **Decompensated cirrhosis with tense ascites** (SBP risk, encephalopathy, GI bleed) → urgent assessment, diagnostic paracentesis if ascites + sepsis features

Immediate actions if red flags

- ABCDE; oxygen if hypoxic; IV access
- ECG if cardiac/renal concern; urgent imaging if VTE suspected
- Treat sepsis/anaphylaxis immediately where indicated

B — Bedside assessment (focused history and exam)

Focused history

Clarify pattern

- **Onset/time course:** sudden vs gradual; episodic; progression
- **Distribution: unilateral vs bilateral**, legs vs generalized, facial/periorbital (renal), abdominal distension (ascites)
- **Associated symptoms**
    - **HF:** dyspnoea, orthopnoea/PND, reduced exercise tolerance
    - **Renal/nephrotic:** frothy urine, reduced urine output
    - **Liver:** jaundice, pruritus, bruising, alcohol history
    - **DVT:** calf pain, recent immobility/surgery, malignancy, OCP/pregnancy
    - **Hypothyroid:** weight gain, cold intolerance, constipation
- **Medication causes:** dihydropyridine CCBs (amlodipine), NSAIDs, steroids, thiazolidinediones, gabapentin/pregabalin, oestrogens
- **PMH:** HF/IHD, CKD, liver disease, VTE, cancer, pregnancy, sleep apnoea
- **Fluid/salt intake**, recent IV fluids

Focused exam

- **General:** weight, BP, pallor, jaundice, cachexia
- **Volume status:** JVP, mucous membranes, postural BP
- **Cardiorespiratory:** crackles, S3, murmurs, hepatomegaly
- **Abdominal:** ascites, liver stigmata
- **Leg exam:** pitting vs non-pitting, warmth/erythema,

tenderness, calf circumference, varicose veins
- **Skin/lymph:** chronic venous changes, eczema, lymphoedema (non-pitting, "stemmer sign")
- **Urine dip** at bedside if possible

C-Core investigations (workup)

Baseline tests (most new/unexplained edema)
- **FBC**
- **U&E/creatinine** (renal function), electrolytes
- **LFTs** + **albumin**
- **Urine dip** + **ACR/PCR** (proteinuria), ± MSU if infection suspected
- **TSH** (if features suggest hypothyroidism)
- **ECG**
- Consider **BNP/NT-proBNP** if HF suspected

Targeted tests

If heart failure suspected
- **CXR** (congestion/effusions)
- **Echocardiography** (LV function/valves)
- BNP helps rule out if low (context-dependent)

If nephrotic syndrome / renal cause suspected
- Quantify protein: **ACR/PCR** ± 24h protein (if needed)
- Serum albumin, lipids; consider renal ultrasound if AKI/obstruction
- Autoimmune screen only if clinically indicated (e.g., ANA, complements)

If liver disease / portal HTN suspected

- LFTs, INR, albumin; **USS liver** with portal/hepatic flow as indicated
- If ascites: **diagnostic paracentesis** (SAAG, albumin, cell count, culture) when appropriate

If DVT suspected (unilateral)

- **Wells score** → **D-dimer** (if appropriate) → **compression Doppler ultrasound**
- If PE symptoms: CTPA per pathway

If chronic venous insufficiency/lymphoedema suspected

- Often clinical; duplex venous ultrasound if uncertain or to plan management

📋 Mnemonic for Common and Serious Causes of edema: "HEARTS FAIL"

H Heart failure, where raised venous pressure from right-sided or congestive failure causes dependent swelling.

E End-stage renal disease or nephrotic syndrome, where sodium and water retention and protein loss lead to generalised oedema.

A Allergy or angioedema, caused by capillary leakage due to histamine release.

R Renal failure, acute or chronic, where fluid retention occurs secondary to impaired excretion.

T Thrombosis, particularly deep vein thrombosis (DVT), producing painful, unilateral swelling.

S Salt excess or drug-induced oedema, seen with NSAIDs, calcium channel blockers, or corticosteroids.

F   Failure of the liver (cirrhosis), where hypoalbuminemia and portal hypertension contribute to ascites and leg oedema.

A   Anaemia or hypoalbuminemia, from malnutrition or protein-losing states.

I   Infection or inflammation, such as cellulitis causing localised swelling and erythema.

L   Lymphatic obstruction or malignancy, such as lymphoma or postoperative lymphoedema.

An easy way to remember it: *"HEARTS FAIL when fluid can't drain — Heart, Kidney, Liver, Lymph, and Drugs remain."*

Mnemonic for Red Flags of edema: "SWELL FAST"

S   Sudden onset oedema, which may indicate DVT, acute heart failure, acute renal failure, or anaphylaxis.

W   Worsening shortness of breath or orthopnoea, raising concern for congestive cardiac failure or pulmonary oedema.

E   Early morning facial or periorbital swelling, a classic feature of nephrotic syndrome or renal disease.

L   Low urine output (oliguria), suggestive of acute kidney injury or fluid overload.

L   Liver stigmata, ascites, or jaundice, pointing to hepatic cirrhosis or portal hypertension.

F   Facial or airway swelling with rash or hypotension, an emergency sign of anaphylaxis or angioedema.

A   Asymmetrical, painful unilateral swelling, usually due to DVT or cellulitis.

S   Swelling with weight loss or lymphadenopathy, which can indicate malignancy or lymphatic obstruction.

T Tense oedema in pregnancy, especially facial or hand swelling with headache or visual symptoms, warning of pre-eclampsia or HELLP syndrome.

An easy way to remember: *"SWELL FAST — if oedema appears suddenly or spreads rapidly, think systemic or sinister."*

Fever

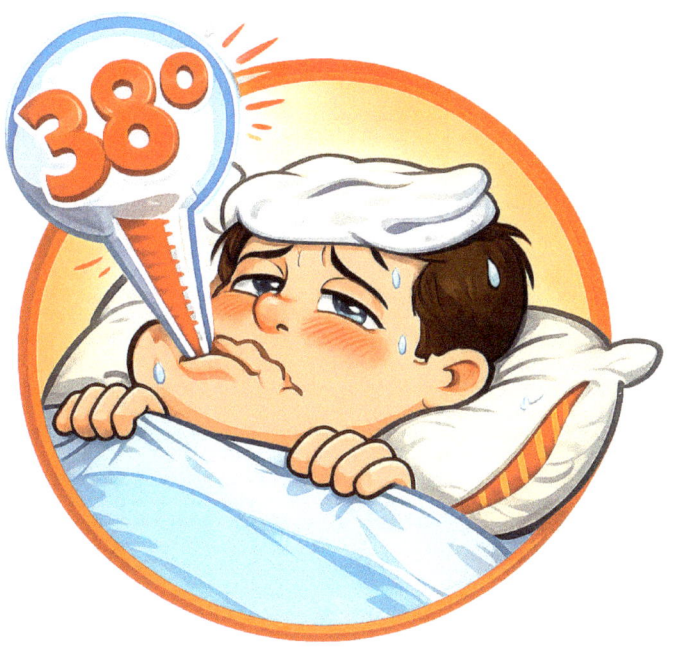

Red Flags: Fever

- ⚠ Fever with hypotension, tachycardia, or confusion
- ⚠ Fever with neck stiffness, photophobia, or altered consciousness
- ⚠ Fever with rash, petechiae, or purpura
- ⚠ Fever with rigors, jaundice, or right upper quadrant pain
- ⚠ Fever with productive cough, pleuritic pain, or breathlessness
- ⚠ Fever with back pain, focal tenderness, or neurological deficit
- ⚠ Fever with severe headache, jaw claudication, or visual symptoms (in elderly)
- ⚠ Fever with recent travel, especially to tropical regions
- ⚠ Fever with night sweats, weight loss, or lymphadenopathy
- ⚠ Fever with new-onset arthritis, rash, or multiorgan involvement
- ⚠ Fever in immunocompromised or neutropenic patient
- ⚠ Neutropenia

∏ **Fever with hypotension, tachycardia, or confusion:**
- ❖ **Implications / Diagnoses:** Sepsis or septic shock, Bacteraemia (e.g. pneumonia, pyelonephritis, meningitis):

- ❖ **Investigations:** Full sepsis screen: FBC, CRP, blood cultures (×2), urine culture, Chest X-ray, urinalysis, stool cultures (if indicated), Lactate, renal & liver function tests, Early warning score (NEWS2), blood pressure, ECG.

∏ Fever with neck stiffness, photophobia, or altered consciousness:

- ❖ **Implications/Diagnoses:** Meningitis or meningoencephalitis.
- ❖ **Investigations:** Urgent lumbar puncture (after CT if raised ICP suspected), CSF analysis: cell count, protein, glucose, Gram stain, culture, PCR, Blood cultures, FBC, CRP, CT or MRI brain (if focal neurology or reduced GCS).

∏ Fever with new murmur or cardiac symptoms:

- ❖ **Implications / Diagnoses:** Infective endocarditis.
- ❖ **Investigations:** Blood cultures (3 sets from different sites before antibiotics), Echocardiography (transthoracic ± transoesophageal), FBC, ESR, CRP, renal profile, Urinalysis (microscopic haematuria), ECG.

∏ Fever with rash, petechiae, or purpura:

- ❖ **Implications / Diagnoses:** Meningococcaemia, septicaemia, toxic shock syndrome, vasculitis, or drug reaction.
- ❖ **Investigations:** Full sepsis screen (blood, urine cultures), FBC, coagulation profile, LFTs, renal function, Blood film (schistocytes for DIC), inflammatory markers, Skin swabs or biopsy if vasculitis suspected.

∏ Fever with rigors, jaundice, or right upper quadrant pain:

- ❖ **Implications / Diagnoses:** Ascending cholangitis (Charcot's triad), Liver abscess / biliary sepsis.
- ❖ **Investigations:** LFTs (ALP, GGT, bilirubin), Abdominal ultrasound or CT (biliary dilatation, abscess), Blood cultures, FBC, CRP, Coagulation profile, renal function.

∏ Fever with productive cough, pleuritic pain, or breathlessness:
- **Implications / Diagnoses:** Pneumonia / lung abscess / pulmonary embolism (with infarction)
- **Investigations:** Chest X-ray, Sputum culture, blood cultures, Arterial blood gas (if hypoxic), CRP, WCC, CT pulmonary angiography if PE suspected.

∏ Fever with back pain, focal tenderness, or neurological deficit:
- **Implications / Diagnoses:** Spinal epidural abscess, osteomyelitis, or pyelonephritis.
- **Investigations:** MRI spine (if neurological signs or midline tenderness), Blood cultures, urine culture, ESR, CRP, FBC, CT or ultrasound for renal tract if pyelonephritis suspected.

∏ Fever with severe headache, jaw claudication, or visual symptoms (in elderly):
- **Implications / Diagnoses:** Giant cell arteritis (temporal arteritis).
- **Investigations:** ESR, CRP (markedly elevated), Temporal artery biopsy, FBC (normocytic anaemia, thrombocytosis).

∏ Fever with recent travel, especially to tropical regions:
- **Implications / Diagnoses:** Malaria, typhoid, dengue, COVID-19, viral haemorrhagic fevers
- **Investigations:** Thick and thin blood films for malaria (repeat ×3 over 48h), Blood cultures, LFTs, renal function, Dengue/typhoid serology, PCR if available, Full travel and vaccination history.

∏ Fever with night sweats, weight loss, or lymphadenopathy:
- **Implications / Diagnoses:** Malignancy (lymphoma, leukaemia), Tuberculosis (TB), Endocarditis (subacute).

- ❖ **Investigations:** FBC, ESR, CRP, Blood cultures (for subacute infections), CXR, QuantiFERON-TB or Mantoux, CT chest/abdomen/pelvis, lymph node biopsy if indicated.

⊓ Fever with new-onset arthritis, rash, or multiorgan involvement:

- ❖ **Implications / Diagnoses:** Systemic autoimmune disease (SLE, vasculitis, Still's disease).
- ❖ **Investigations:** ANA, dsDNA, ANCA, complement levels, ESR, CRP, urinalysis (protein/haematuria), Joint aspiration if septic arthritis suspected.

⊓ Fever in immunocompromised or neutropenic patient:

- ❖ **Implications / Diagnoses:** Neutropenic sepsis, opportunistic infections, fungal sepsis.
- ❖ **Investigations:** Urgent FBC (neutrophil count), CRP, Blood cultures (including fungal), CXR, urine and sputum cultures, Consider early broad-spectrum antibiotics as per neutropenic sepsis protocol

🗝 Key Points:

- Fever can be caused by – infectious (most common), neoplastic/malignancy, and inflammatory (rheumatic, non rheumatic and drug related).
- Pyrexia of unknown origin is defined as > 38.3 C with no identified cause after 3 days of inpatient hospital investigations or > 3 outpatient visits.

ABC approach to fever (evaluation + workup)

A — Assessment and immediate threats

Rapid severity check (treat sepsis until proven otherwise if unwell)

- Obs/NEWS2: **RR, SpO$_2$, HR, BP, temp, GCS/AVPU**
- Check **capillary glucose**, urine output, hydration, rash, rigors.
- Identify **septic shock**: hypotension, lactate raised, mottling, oliguria, confusion.

Immediate threats / red flags (urgent same-day / ED)

- **Sepsis / septic shock**
- **Meningitis/encephalitis:** headache, neck stiffness, photophobia, seizures, rash, reduced GCS
- **Neutropenic sepsis** (chemo, haematological malignancy, transplant, high-dose steroids)
- **Severe malaria** (fever + travel to endemic area)
- **Endocarditis:** persistent fever + murmur, embolic phenomena, IVDU, prosthetic valve
- **Toxic shock / necrotising soft tissue infection:** severe pain out of proportion, rapidly spreading erythema, hypotension
- **Heat illness** (hyperthermia with altered mental state)

Immediate actions if any red flags

- **Sepsis 6** (within 1 hour where indicated): O$_2$, IV fluids, IV antibiotics, blood cultures, lactate, urine output monitoring

- Early senior review; isolate if high-risk infection suspected (e.g., meningococcal, viral haemorrhagic risk, TB)
- If meningitis/encephalitis suspected: give **empirical IV antibiotics** ± **acyclovir** per local pathway (don't delay for LP if unstable)

B — Bedside assessment (focused history and exam)

Focused history (source + risk factors)

- **Timeline:** onset, pattern (intermittent/continuous), rigors, night sweats
- **Symptoms by system:**
    - Respiratory (cough, dyspnoea, pleuritic pain)
    - Urinary (dysuria, flank pain)
    - GI (diarrhoea, RUQ pain)
    - Skin/soft tissue (wounds, cellulitis, bites)
    - Neuro (headache, photophobia, confusion)
    - MSK (hot joint/back pain)
- **Exposures:** sick contacts, recent travel, animals, ticks, food/water, occupation, recent procedures/dental work
- **Devices:** IV lines, urinary catheter, prosthetic joints/valves, pacemaker
- **Immunosuppression:** chemo, steroids, HIV risk, asplenia
- **Drug fever** (new meds), recent antibiotics (C. diff risk)
- **Thrombo/inflammatory clues:** pleuritic pain (PE), temporal headache/jaw claudication (GCA), autoimmune symptoms

Focused exam

- Full set of obs + hydration/perfusion

- **Skin:** rashes (non-blanching?), cellulitis, lines, pressure sores
- **ENT:** throat/ears/sinuses
- **Chest:** crackles/focal signs
- **CVS:** new murmur, peripheral stigmata of endocarditis
- **Abdomen:** RUQ tenderness, suprapubic/CVA tenderness
- **Neuro:** meningism, focal deficit, delirium screen
- **Joints/spine:** hot swollen joint, vertebral tenderness (discitis/SEA red flag)

C- Core investigations (workup)

Baseline for most significant fever (especially if admitted)

- **Bloods: FBC, U&E/creatinine, LFT, CRP (± ESR), glucose**
- **Lactate** (VBG/ABG) if unwell or sepsis suspected
- **Blood cultures** (ideally before antibiotics) if systemic features
- **Urinalysis ± urine culture**
- **CXR** if any respiratory symptoms/signs or no clear source

Targeted microbiology (based on clues)

- **Sputum culture** if productive cough; viral PCR in season/outbreak
- **Stool culture/C. diff** if diarrhoea (esp. post-antibiotics)
- **Swabs** from wounds/line sites; remove/replace suspected infected lines per policy
- **Malaria film/rapid test** for fever with travel to endemic regions (even if months ago)

Imaging / procedures (source control)

- **Ultrasound** RUQ if biliary source; renal US if obstruction suspected
- **CT chest/abdomen/pelvis** if persistent fever with unclear source, severe abdominal signs, or concern for deep infection
- **LP** if meningitis/encephalitis suspected (after CT if indicated)
- **Echocardiography** (TTE ± TOE) if **endocarditis** suspected
- **Joint aspiration** for hot swollen joint (cell count, crystals, Gram stain/culture)
- **MRI spine** if back pain + fever + neuro symptoms (epidural abscess/discitis)

Mnemonic for Fever Red Flags: "HOT ALERT"

H – Hypotension / tachycardia / confusion → Sepsis

O – Organ dysfunction (renal, hepatic, respiratory) → Sepsis / MODS

T – Travel history → Malaria, Typhoid, Dengue

A – Altered consciousness / meningism → Meningitis / Encephalitis

L – Lymphadenopathy / weight loss → TB / Lymphoma

E – Endocarditis signs (new murmur) → Infective endocarditis

R – Rash / petechiae / purpura → Meningococcaemia / Sepsis

T – Tender RUQ or back pain → Cholangitis / Abscess / Spinal sepsis

Falls

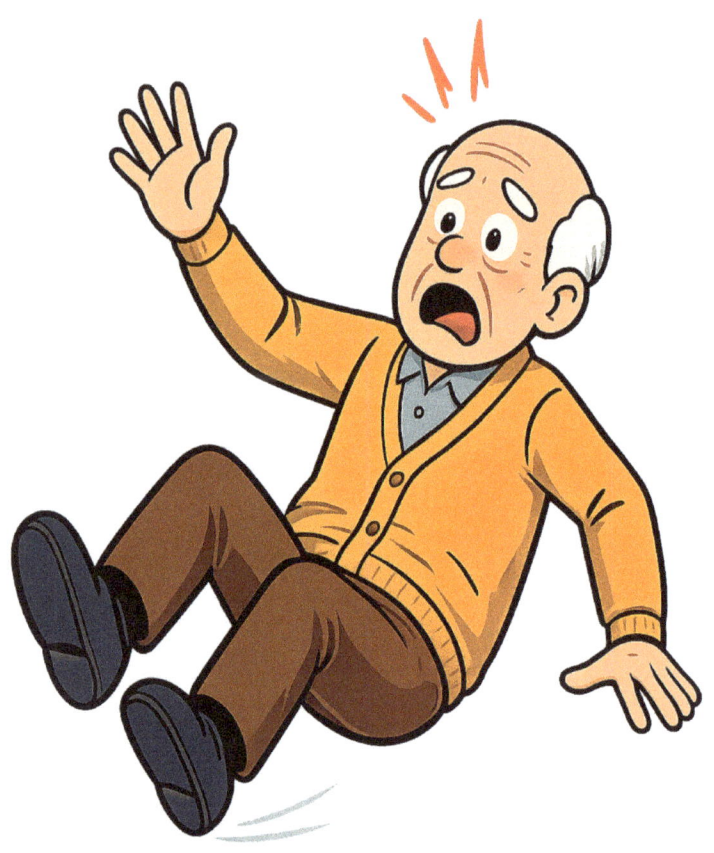

Red Flags: Falls

- Loss of Consciousness Before or During Fall
- Head Injury or Loss of Consciousness After Fall
- New Neurological Symptoms
- Sudden Collapse Without Warning
- Palpitations, Chest Pain, or Dyspnoea Before Fall
- Incontinence, Weakness, or Severe Back Pain
- Severe Pain or Limb/Spine Deformity After Fall
- Fall While on Anticoagulation or Bleeding Disorder
- Recurrent Unexplained Falls
- Gait Disturbance, Tremor, or Parkinsonism
- Systemic Symptoms (Fever, Weight Loss, Night Sweats)
- Visual or Balance Disturbance Before Fall

Loss of Consciousness Before or During Fall:

- **Implications / Diagnoses:** Suggests a syncopal or neurological event rather than a mechanical fall. Causes include cardiac syncope (arrhythmias, structural heart disease), vasovagal syncope, orthostatic hypotension, and seizures.
- **Investigations:** ECG, 24-hour Holter/telemetry, echocardiogram, lying and standing BP, blood glucose, and EEG if seizure suspected.

∏ Head Injury or Loss of Consciousness After Fall:
- ❖ **Implications / Diagnoses:** May indicate intracranial haemorrhage (subdural, extradural, intracerebral) or concussion, particularly in older adults or those on anticoagulants.
- ❖ **Investigations:** Urgent CT head (NICE criteria), neurological, observations, and GCS monitoring.

∏ New Neurological Symptoms:
- ❖ **Implications / Diagnoses:** Focal deficits, confusion, or slurred speech suggest stroke, TIA, or subdural haematoma.
- ❖ **Investigations:** CT or MRI brain, FBC, U&E, CRP, ECG, and carotid Doppler where appropriate.

∏ Sudden Collapse Without Warning:
- ❖ **Implications / Diagnoses:** Suggests cardiac arrhythmia (heart block, VT/VF), aortic stenosis, hypertrophic cardiomyopathy, or massive pulmonary embolism.
- ❖ **Investigations:** ECG, cardiac telemetry, troponin, echocardiogram, D-dimer or CTPA if PE suspected.

∏ Palpitations, Chest Pain, or Dyspnoea Before Fall:
- ❖ **Implications / Diagnoses:** Indicates arrhythmia, acute coronary syndrome, or pulmonary embolism.
- ❖ **Investigations:** ECG, cardiac enzymes, chest X-ray, and echocardiogram or CTPA as indicated.

∏ Incontinence, Weakness, or Severe Back Pain:
- ❖ **Implications / Diagnoses:** Suggests cauda equina syndrome or spinal cord compression, often due to disc prolapse or malignancy.
- ❖ **Investigations:** Urgent MRI spine, neurological exam, and post-void bladder scan.

∏ Severe Pain or Limb/Spine Deformity After Fall:

- **Implications / Diagnoses:** Suggests fracture (neck of femur, pelvis, vertebra, wrist).
- **Investigations:** X-ray of affected region; CT if inconclusive.

∏ Fall While on Anticoagulation or Bleeding Disorder:

- **Implications / Diagnoses:** High risk of **intracranial or internal bleeding**, even if asymptomatic.
- **Investigations:** Urgent CT head, FBC, coagulation profile.

∏ Recurrent Unexplained Falls:

- **Implications / Diagnoses:** May be due to arrhythmias, postural hypotension, or medication effects (antihypertensives, sedatives, hypoglycaemics).
- **Investigations:** Medication review, lying & standing BP, ECG, blood glucose.

∏ Gait Disturbance, Tremor, or Parkinsonism:

- **Implications / Diagnoses:** Suggests Parkinson's disease, cerebellar disease, or normal pressure hydrocephalus.
- **Investigations:** Neurological exam, MRI brain, review for dopamine-blocking medications.

∏ Systemic Symptoms (Fever, Weight Loss, Night Sweats):

- **Implications / Diagnoses:** Suggests malignancy (bone mets) or systemic infection (sepsis, endocarditis).
- **Investigations:** FBC, CRP, ESR, chest X-ray, blood cultures, CT/MRI as required.

∏ Visual or Balance Disturbance Before Fall:

- **Implications / Diagnoses:** May reflect vestibular dysfunction, visual impairment, or vertebrobasilar insufficiency.
- **Investigations:** ENT/ophthalmology review, MRI/MRA brain, carotid Doppler, postural BP.

🗝️ Key points:

Key History Points (4 P's)

- **Pre-fall:** dizziness, chest pain, palpitations, visual disturbance
- **Peri-fall:** witnessed movements, LOC, posture, seizure activity
- **Post-fall:** confusion, injury, duration until recovery
- **Previous falls:** pattern suggests underlying cause

Define the Event

- Determine: *Is it a fall, syncope, mechanical trip, or collapse?*
- Ask about **witnessed features**, prodrome (dizziness, chest pain, palpitations), and recovery time.

Common Causes

- **Cardiovascular:** orthostatic hypotension, arrhythmias, aortic stenosis
- **Neurological:** Parkinsonism, stroke/TIA, peripheral neuropathy
- **Medications:** antihypertensives, sedatives, antipsychotics, alcohol
- **Musculoskeletal/Functional:** frailty, poor mobility, sarcopenia
- **Environmental:** poor lighting, loose rugs, footwear

ABC approach to fall (evaluation + workup):

A — Assessment and immediate threats

Rapid severity check (ABCDE)

- Obs/NEWS2, pain score, glucose, conscious level.

- Assume **c-spine** risk if significant head/neck trauma or reduced GCS.

Immediate threats / red flags (urgent ED / senior review)

- **Head injury / intracranial bleed:** reduced GCS, persistent vomiting, severe headache, seizure, new focal neurology, **on anticoagulants/antiplatelets**
- **C-spine injury:** neck pain, neuro deficit, high-energy mechanism
- **Major haemorrhage:** hypotension, tachycardia, pallor; pelvic/long-bone injury
- **Hip fracture:** unable to weight bear, shortened/external rotation, severe groin pain
- **Sepsis** as precipitant (fever, hypotension, confusion)
- **ACS/arrhythmia/syncope:** chest pain, palpitations, exertional syncope, family history sudden death
- **Stroke/TIA:** focal deficits, new gait/coordination change
- **Hypoglycaemia** or severe electrolyte disturbance
- **Safeguarding:** unexplained injuries, neglect, domestic violence risk

Immediate actions

- Analgesia early; immobilise if suspected fracture/spine injury
- If head injury risk: urgent **CT head** per pathway (and C-spine imaging if indicated)
- If hip fracture suspected: urgent **pelvic/hip X-ray** (and femur if needed), early orthogeriatrics/ortho
- If syncope suspected: **ECG**, postural BP, treat reversible causes

B — Bedside assessment (focused history and exam)

Focused history (what caused the fall?)

- **Mechanism:** trip/slip vs collapse; witnessed? head strike? loss of consciousness?
- **Prodrome:** dizziness, palpitations, chest pain, breathlessness, visual change, aura, nausea
- **Post-event:** confusion, tongue bite, incontinence (seizure); duration on floor (rhabdo risk)
- **Injuries/pain:** head/neck, hip, wrist, back
- **Baseline:** mobility, falls history, frailty, cognition, continence, vision/hearing
- **Meds:** antihypertensives, diuretics, sedatives/benzos, opioids, antidepressants, hypoglycaemics; **anticoagulants**
- **Triggers:** infection, dehydration, missed meals, alcohol, new environment
- **Functional/safeguarding:** home hazards, footwear, support at home

Focused exam

- **Neuro:** GCS, pupils, focal deficit, gait if safe
- **Cardio:** pulse (rate/rhythm), murmurs, signs of HF; **postural BP**
- **Resp:** hypoxia, infection signs
- **MSK:** inspect/palpate spine, pelvis, hips; limb deformity; ROM cautiously
- **Skin:** bruising pattern, pressure sores; hydration
- **Bedside:** glucose; consider bladder scan if retention contributes

C- Core investigations (workup)
Core tests for most medical falls (especially older adults)
- **ECG** (arrhythmia, ischemia, conduction block)
- **Bloods: FBC, U&E/creatinine**, glucose, **CRP** (if infection suspected)
- **CK** if prolonged time on floor / muscle pain (rhabdomyolysis)
- **Troponin** if chest pain/ECG changes or collapse suspicious for ACS
- **Urinalysis** ± culture (if urinary symptoms or delirium features)
- Consider **orthostatic vitals** documented properly

Imaging (based on presentation)
- **CT head** if head injury risk factors (anticoagulation, LOC/amnesia, neuro signs, persistent headache/vomiting, frailty) per local rule
- **CT C-spine** if neck pain, neuro deficit, or high-risk mechanism
- **X-ray hip/pelvis** if pain or inability to weight bear; **X-ray wrist/forearm** if FOOSH injury
- **CXR** if respiratory symptoms or sepsis source unclear

Further tests if indicated
- **Telemetry/Holter** if intermittent arrhythmia suspected
- **Echo** if murmur/structural heart disease suspected
- **B12/folate, TSH, vitamin D** in recurrent falls/frailty workup (non-urgent)
- **Falls MDT** assessment: physio gait/balance, OT home hazards, vision/hearing review, medication rationalisation

Mnemonic: **FALLSCHECK**

Letter	Meaning	Use
F	**F**requency of falls	One-off vs recurrent suggests underlying cause
A	**A**ntecedents (what happened before)	Dizziness, chest pain, palpitations, vision changes
L	**L**oss of consciousness	Suggests syncope or seizure
L	**L**ocation & environment	Home hazards, poor lighting, slippery floor
S	**S**hoes & mobility aids	Poor footwear or incorrect aid increases risk
C	**C**ardiac causes	Check pulse, murmurs, arrhythmia symptoms
H	**H**ypotension (lying & standing BP)	Orthostatic hypotension is common cause
E	**E**yesight & sensory issues	Cataracts, poor acuity, neuropathy
C	**C**ognition & confusion	Dementia, delirium, post-ictal state
K	**K**nock (injuries & complications)	Head injury, fractures, especially on anticoagulants

✅ Summary

Red flags in falls should prompt a **systematic multisystem evaluation**.

- **Cardiac:** ECG, Holter, Echo, Troponin, CTPA
- **Neurological:** CT/MRI brain/spine, EEG
- **Metabolic:** U&E, Glucose, Calcium, B12, Vitamin D
- **Musculoskeletal:** X-ray or DEXA
- **General:** Medication review, Lying/standing BP, Vision and gait assessment.

Gastrointestinal bleeding

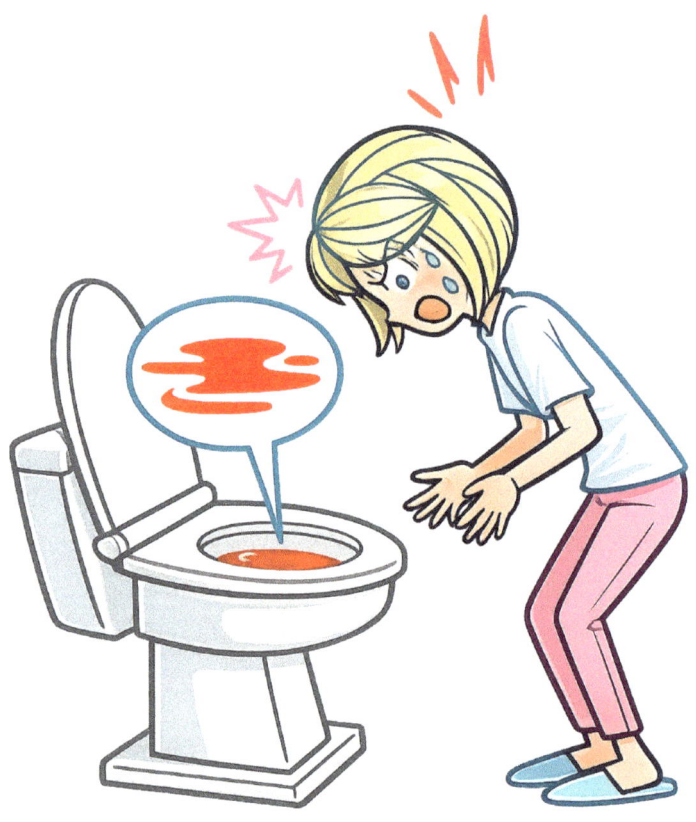

Red Flags: Gastrointestinal bleeding

- ⚠ Haematemesis (vomiting blood or coffee-ground vomitus)
- ⚠ Haemodynamic instability (hypotension, tachycardia, syncope, shock)
- ⚠ Malaena (black tarry stools) or bright red rectal bleeding (haematochezia)
- ⚠ History of liver disease, alcohol abuse, or stigmata of chronic liver disease
- ⚠ Use of NSAIDs, aspirin, steroids, or anticoagulants
- ⚠ Weight loss, anorexia, or iron-deficiency anaemia with occult blood
- ⚠ Recurrent or persistent minor bleeding
- ⚠ Abdominal pain, tenderness, or peritonism
- ⚠ Fever or rigors with bleeding
- ⚠ Bleeding in elderly or comorbid patient
- ⚠ Recurrent or persistent minor bleeding
- ⚠ Abdominal pain, tenderness, or peritonism
- ⚠ Fever or rigors with bleeding
- ⚠ GI bleeding in a young adult with family history of bowel disease

∏ **Haematemesis (vomiting blood or coffee-ground vomitus):**
- ❖ **Implications / Diagnoses: Upper GI bleed** from peptic ulcer, varices, Mallory-Weiss tear, erosive gastritis, or malignancy. **Massive haematemesis** suggests variceal rupture or arterial ulcer erosion.

- ❖ **Investigations:** Urgent FBC, U&E, LFTs, coagulation profile, blood group and cross-match, Endoscopy (OGD) within 24 h (sooner if unstable),Naso-gastric aspirate may confirm upper source if unclear., Liver screen and ultrasound if varices suspected.

∏ Haemodynamic instability (hypotension, tachycardia, syncope, shock):

- ❖ **Implications / Diagnoses: Massive or ongoing bleed** — can occur with either upper or lower GI source. Suggests hypovolaemic shock, potentially fatal if untreated.
- ❖ **Investigations:** Immediate ABC resuscitation with IV access ×2, fluids ± blood transfusion. Serial FBC, lactate, and cross-match. Endoscopy / colonoscopy / CT angiography once stable. Monitor urine output and vital signs closely.

∏ Malaena (black tarry stools) or bright red rectal bleeding (haematochezia):

- ❖ **Implications / Diagnoses:** Melaena → usually upper GI source (peptic ulcer, varices). Haematochezia → lower GI source (diverticulosis, malignancy, angiodysplasia, IBD) or massive upper bleed with rapid transit.
- ❖ **Investigations:** OGD first if haemodynamically unstable (upper source more likely). Colonoscopy if stable or upper source excluded. FBC, ferritin, coagulation profile. CT angiography / tagged RBC scan if bleeding site uncertain.

∏ History of liver disease, alcohol abuse, or stigmata of chronic liver disease:

- ❖ **Implications / Diagnoses:** Oesophageal or gastric varices, portal hypertensive gastropathy. Coagulopathy from hepatic failure worsening bleeding risk.

- ❖ **Investigations:** LFTs, albumin, INR, and platelet count., Abdominal ultrasound with Doppler for portal hypertension. Urgent OGD for variceal assessment.

∏ Use of NSAIDs, aspirin, steroids, or anticoagulants:

- ❖ **Implications / Diagnoses:** Peptic ulcer disease, erosive gastritis, or drug-exacerbated bleeding. Anticoagulant-associated haemorrhage can be severe even with small lesions.
- ❖ **Investigations:** Medication review, INR / PT / aPTT., OGD to identify source. Helicobacter pylori testing if ulcer suspected.

∏ Weight loss, anorexia, or iron-deficiency anaemia with occult blood:

- ❖ **Implications / Diagnoses:** Gastrointestinal malignancy (gastric, duodenal, or colorectal cancer).
- ❖ **Investigations:** FBC, ferritin, faecal occult blood or FIT test, OGD + colonoscopy (bidirectional endoscopy), CT abdomen / pelvis for staging if tumour suspected.

∏ Recurrent or persistent minor bleeding:

- ❖ **Implications / Diagnoses:** Angiodysplasia, malignancy, polyps, inflammatory bowel disease, or Dieulafoy lesion.
- ❖ **Investigations:** Endoscopy / colonoscopy, ± capsule endoscopy for small bowel, CT angiography if ongoing bleeding with negative endoscopy.

∏ Abdominal pain, tenderness, or peritonism:

- ❖ **Implications / Diagnoses:** Perforated ulcer, ischaemic bowel, or inflammatory bowel disease. Pain + bleeding often implies ulcer erosion or infarction.
- ❖ **Investigations:** Erect chest X-ray (free air under diaphragm), CT abdomen for perforation or ischaemia, Amylase, lactate, LFTs.

∏ Fever or rigors with bleeding:

- ❖ **Implications / Diagnoses:** Infectious colitis, liver abscess, bacteraemia secondary to variceal bleeding, or sepsis from bowel ischaemia.
- ❖ **Investigations:** FBC, CRP, blood cultures, stool cultures., CT abdomen to exclude abscess or ischaemic colitis.

∏ Bleeding in elderly or comorbid patient:

- ❖ **Implications / Diagnoses:** Malignancy, angiodysplasia, ischaemic colitis, or polypharmacy-related bleeding, High risk for shock and anaemia even with smaller bleeds.
- ❖ **Investigations:** OGD and colonoscopy (full evaluation)., FBC, ferritin, renal function, and coagulation profile., CT angiography if endoscopy negative.

∏ GI bleeding in a young adult with family history of bowel disease:

- ❖ **Implications / Diagnoses:** Inflammatory bowel disease, polyposis syndromes, or Meckel's diverticulum.
- ❖ **Investigations:** Faecal calprotectin, stool cultures, colonoscopy ± biopsy, Technetium-99m Meckel's scan in children.

🗝 Key Points:

- Bleeding of any cause is potentially more severe and more frequently in patients with chronic liver disease(e.g chronic alcohol abuse, chronic hepatitis), in those with coagulation disorders or in those taking certain drugs (heparin, warfarin, NSAIDs, clopidogrel, SSRIs.
- Rectal bleeding may result from upper or lower GI bleeding.

- The most common cause of major bleeding are Peptic ulcer, Diverticular disease and Angiodysplasia and variceal bleeding.
- GI bleeding stops spontaneously in 80% of patients.

ABC approach to gastrointestinal bleeding (evaluation + workup):

A — Assessment and immediate threats

Rapid severity check (ABCDE)

- Obs/NEWS2: **HR, BP, RR, SpO$_2$, temp, GCS**
- Look for **shock:** hypotension, tachycardia, cool peripheries, syncope, confusion, oliguria.
- Identify bleed type: **haematemesis/coffee-ground** (upper), **melaena** (upper), **fresh PR blood** (usually lower but can be brisk upper).

Immediate threats / red flags (urgent resus / senior help)

- **Haemodynamic instability** or ongoing large-volume bleeding
- **Massive haematemesis** / inability to protect airway
- **Significant comorbidity** (IHD, HF, CKD, cirrhosis), **elderly/frail**
- **Anticoagulants/antiplatelets** (warfarin/DOACs), known coagulopathy
- **Cirrhosis/portal HTN** → possible **variceal bleed**
- **Ongoing chest pain / ischaemia** (demand MI)

Immediate actions (do now)

- **Call for help early** (senior/anaesthetics/endoscopy/ICU if unstable)

- 2 large-bore IVs, bloods, **group & save/crossmatch**
- **Resuscitate with fluids/blood** as per major haemorrhage protocol
- **Restrictive transfusion** often used (target Hb ~70–90 g/L; higher if active IHD—follow local policy)
- **Reversal/haemostasis support** if indicated:
  - Warfarin: vitamin K + PCC per protocol
  - DOAC: specific reversal where available / PCC per pathway
  - Platelets/FFP guided by labs/bleeding risk
- **Upper GI bleed suspected:** keep **NBM**, antiemetic, consider **PPI**; if **variceal suspected** start **terlipressin + IV antibiotics** per local pathway
- **Airway:** intubation consideration if massive haematemesis/low GCS

B — Bedside assessment (focused history and exam)

Focused history

- **Bleed description:** haematemesis (fresh vs coffee-ground), melaena, maroon PR blood, clots, frequency, estimated volume
- **Symptoms of hypovolaemia:** dizziness, syncope, chest pain, breathlessness
- **Upper GI clues:** epigastric pain, reflux, retching (Mallory–Weiss)
- **Lower GI clues:** change in bowel habit, abdominal cramps, diarrhoea, IBD, diverticular disease
- **Liver disease/portal HTN:** jaundice, ascites, varices, alcohol history

- **Medication:** NSAIDs, aspirin, steroids, SSRIs; anticoagulants/antiplatelets
- **Past history:** prior GI bleed, ulcer disease, known varices, cancer, CKD
- **Infection/ischaemia clues:** severe abdo pain, vascular disease (ischaemic colitis)

Focused exam

- **General:** pallor, diaphoresis, cap refill, mental state
- **Abdominal:** tenderness, peritonism, masses
- **PR exam:** melaena vs fresh blood; mass; haemorrhoids (don't assume haemorrhoids are the cause)
- **Stigmata of chronic liver disease;** ascites
- **CVS/resp:** signs of fluid overload/heart disease (important for resuscitation targets)

C- Core investigations (workup)

Core labs (send early, repeat as needed)

- **FBC** (Hb/platelets)
- **U&E/creatinine** (AKI; urea may rise in upper GI bleed)
- **LFTs**
- **Coagulation** (INR/PT, aPTT, fibrinogen if massive bleed)
- **Group & save + crossmatch**
- **VBG/ABG ± lactate if shocked**
- ± Troponin if chest pain or significant physiological stress

Risk stratification

- **Upper GI bleed:** calculate **Glasgow–Blatchford Score (GBS)** to guide urgency/disposition
- Consider **Rockall** after endoscopy (inpatient risk)

Imaging/endoscopy (guided by stability + suspected source)

Suspected Upper GI bleed

- **Urgent OGD:**
  - Immediately/within hours if unstable or ongoing bleeding (per local policy)
  - Within 24 hours for most admitted UGIB
- If variceal suspected: manage as variceal until proven otherwise + urgent endoscopy
- Suspected Lower GI bleed
- **If unstable/ongoing significant bleeding: CT angiography** to localise active bleeding ± embolisation
- **If stable: colonoscopy** (timing per pathway) after resuscitation and bowel prep
- Consider **flexible sigmoidoscopy** if suspected distal source and rapid assessment needed

Targeted tests (selected cases)

- **Stool tests** if infectious colitis suspected (diarrhoea + fever)
- **Iron studies** if chronic occult bleed/anaemia (not acute priority)

First 15 minutes (any GI bleed) — bullet checklist

- **ABCDE + call for help early** (senior, anaesthetics if massive haematemesis/low GCS; alert endoscopy/radiology early if heavy ongoing bleed).

- **Monitoring:** continuous SpO$_2$, BP, ECG; 2 sets of obs close together; strict urine output (catheter if shocked).
- **2 wide-bore IV cannulas** (or IO/central access if needed).
- **Bloods immediately:** FBC, U&E, LFTs, **coag (INR/PT, APTT ± fibrinogen if major bleed)**, VBG/ABG + **lactate, group & save + crossmatch**.
- **Resuscitate:**
  - Crystalloid bolus if hypotensive while blood arrives; activate **major haemorrhage** protocol if needed.
  - **Restrictive transfusion** strategy when appropriate (commonly Hb trigger ~ 70 g/L; higher target if ACS/major haemorrhage—use local protocol).
- **Stop/review anticoagulants/antiplatelets**; reverse if major bleeding per local policy (e.g., warfarin → vitamin K + PCC; DOAC → reversal strategy/PCC as per pathway).
- **NBM** (likely endoscopy/anaesthetic) + antiemetic; analgesia as needed.
- **If UGIB likely** (haematemesis/coffee-ground/melaena): start **PPI** (local protocol) and plan **OGD**.
- **If variceal bleed possible (known cirrhosis/portal HTN, stigmata):** start **terlipressin + IV antibiotics** and arrange **urgent endoscopy**. (Endoscopy for suspected variceal haemorrhage is typically targeted **within 12 hours once resuscitated**.)
- **Risk assess (helps urgency/disposition):**
  - UGIB: **Glasgow–Blatchford Score**
  - LGIB: shock index / risk score (e.g., Oakland) alongside clinical judgement.

Choosing OGD vs CTA vs Colonoscopy vs Sigmoidoscopy (practical bullets)

Choose OGD (upper endoscopy) when:
- **Haematemesis** or **coffee-ground vomiting**
- **Melaena**
- Suspected UGIB even with **fresh PR bleeding** if very brisk/unstable (UGIB can present this way)
- **Haemodynamic instability** with suspected UGIB → **urgent OGD after resuscitation**
- Most admitted UGIB (once stabilised) → **OGD within 24 hours**
- Suspected **variceal** UGIB → aim ≤**12 hours post-presentation once resuscitated**

Choose CTA (CT angiography) when:
- **Major ongoing LGIB AND haemodynamic instability (or shock index >1 after initial resuscitation)** to localise active bleeding and guide embolisation/surgery.
- Any situation where you need **rapid localisation** of active bleeding before endoscopic/radiologic therapy (especially unstable patients).

Choose Colonoscopy when:
- Suspected **lower GI bleed** and the patient is **haemodynamically stable** after resuscitation.
- Use for diagnosis ± endoscopic therapy **during the admission** (evidence for "very early" colonoscopy improving outcomes is limited, so timing is usually pragmatic—after stabilisation and bowel prep).

Choose Flexible sigmoidoscopy when:

- Bleeding seems **distal** (fresh PR blood, tenesmus, suspected **proctitis/rectal lesion**) and you need **rapid lower-end evaluation**, often with minimal prep.
- Suspected **acute colitis** (IBD flare/infective colitis/ischaemic colitis) where an early limited exam/biopsies may be useful and full prep colonoscopy is not appropriate initially (follow local GI pathway).

Mnemonic for GI Bleeding Red Flags: "BLOOD LOSS"

B – Black stools / haematemesis → Peptic ulcer, varices

L – Low BP or tachycardia → Shock / active bleeding

O – Old age or comorbidities → Malignancy / poor reserve

O – Ongoing NSAID / anticoagulant use → Drug-related ulcer

D – Drop in Hb / iron deficiency / weight loss → Cancer / chronic bleed

L – Liver disease signs / alcohol history → Varices

O – Ongoing or recurrent bleeds → Angiodysplasia / malignancy

S – Severe pain or peritonism → Perforation / ischaemia

S – Sepsis / fever with bleeding → Infective or ischaemic cause

Headache

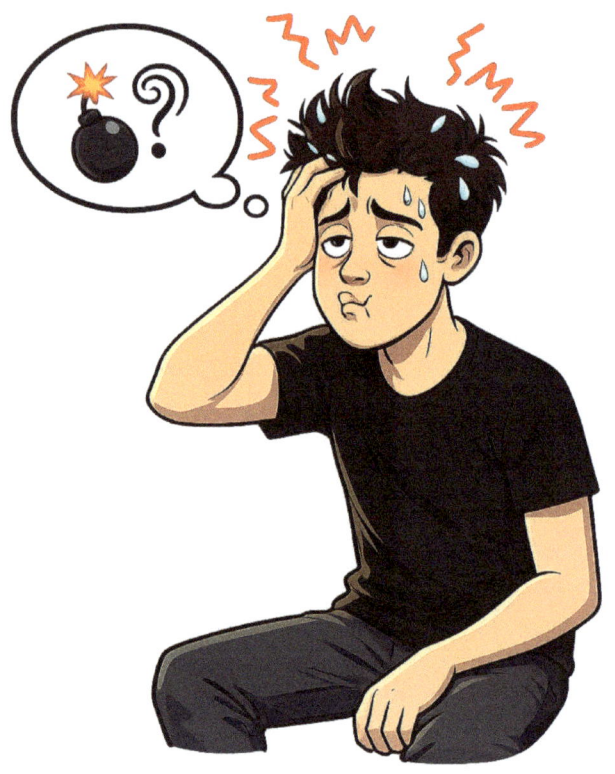

⚑ Red Flags: Headache

- ⚠ Sudden, severe "thunderclap" headache
- ⚠ New onset headache in patients >50 years old
- ⚠ Headache with fever, neck stiffness, photophobia, or altered consciousness
- ⚠ Progressive headache or change in pattern of a known headache
- ⚠ Headache triggered by exertion, coughing, or Valsalva manoeuvre
- ⚠ Headache with neurological deficits, altered mental status or seizures, Papilledema
- ⚠ Headache with visual symptoms (transient loss, double vision, visual aura not typical of migraine)
- ⚠ Headache worse in the morning or with lying down/coughing
- ⚠ Headache after head injury
- ⚠ Headache with systemic features — weight loss, night sweats, malignancy, immunosuppression, pregnancy, or postpartum

∏ **Sudden, severe "thunderclap" headache:**
- ❖ **Implications/diagnoses:** Subarachnoid haemorrhage (SAH), intracerebral haemorrhage, cerebral venous sinus thrombosis.
- ❖ **Investigations:** Urgent non-contrast CT head (within 1 hour if SAH suspected). If CT negative but suspicion high → lumbar puncture after 12 hours (look for xanthochromia). CT or MR venogram if venous sinus thrombosis suspected.

∏ New onset headache in patients >50 years old:

- **Implications/diagnoses:** Giant Cell Arteritis (temporal arteritis), intracranial mass lesion, chronic subdural haematoma.
- **Investigations:** ESR and CRP (usually markedly elevated in GCA), Temporal artery ultrasound or biopsy (confirm GCA), MRI brain to rule out mass lesion or subdural haematoma.

∏ Headache with fever, neck stiffness, photophobia, or altered consciousness:

- **Implications/diagnoses:** Meningitis, encephalitis, brain abscess.
- **Investigations:** Urgent blood cultures, FBC, CRP, Lumbar puncture (after CT head if raised ICP suspected), CSF analysis (cell count, glucose, protein, Gram stain, PCR), MRI brain if abscess or encephalitis suspected.

∏ Progressive headache or change in pattern of a known headache:

- **Implications/diagnoses:** Space-occupying lesion (tumour, abscess), raised intracranial pressure, idiopathic intracranial hypertension.
- **Investigations:** MRI brain with contrast (preferred for intracranial pathology), CT brain if MRI not available, Fundoscopy for papilloedema, Lumbar puncture (opening pressure if no mass lesion on imaging).

∏ Headache triggered by exertion, coughing, or Valsalva manoeuvre:

- **Implications/diagnoses:** Subarachnoid haemorrhage, posterior fossa lesion, Chiari malformation.
- **Investigations:** MRI brain with posterior fossa views, MR angiography if aneurysm suspected.

∏ Headache with neurological deficits, altered mental status or seizures, Papilledema:

- ❖ **Implications/diagnoses:** Stroke, intracranial haemorrhage, venous sinus thrombosis, space-occupying lesion.
- ❖ **Investigations:** Urgent CT or MRI brain, MR angiogram or venogram if vascular cause suspected, EEG if postictal confusion or seizures.

∏ Headache with visual symptoms (transient loss, double vision, visual aura not typical of migraine):

- ❖ **Implications/diagnoses:** Temporal arteritis, intracranial mass, idiopathic intracranial hypertension (IIH), pituitary apoplexy.
- ❖ **Investigations:** Visual fields and fundoscopy (for papilloedema or visual loss), MRI brain and orbits, pituitary MRI if apoplexy suspected., ESR/CRP (for GCA), LP for opening pressure (IIH).

∏ Headache worse in the morning or with lying down/coughing:

- ❖ **Implications/diagnoses:** Raised intracranial pressure (tumour, hydrocephalus, IIH).
- ❖ **Investigations:** MRI brain ± venogram, Fundoscopy for papilloedema, LP (after imaging) for opening pressure.

∏ Headache after head injury:

- ❖ **Implications/diagnoses:** Subdural or extradural haematoma, post-traumatic headache.
- ❖ **Investigations:** CT head (non-contrast) immediately if red flag features (confusion, vomiting, focal neurology), MRI brain for delayed presentations.

∏ Headache with systemic features — weight loss, night sweats, malignancy, immunosuppression, pregnancy, or postpartum:

- ❖ **Implications/diagnoses:** Malignancy with brain metastases, Opportunistic infections (toxoplasmosis, abscess), Cerebral venous sinus thrombosis (postpartum), Preeclampsia/eclampsia.
- ❖ **Investigations: MRI brain ± venogram, Blood tests:** FBC, U&E,
- ❖ LFTs, CRP, autoimmune screen, Urinalysis and BP (for preeclampsia).

🔑 Key points:

- **Immediate or urgent neuroimaging -CT or MRI should be done in patients with any of the following:-** Thunderclap headache, altered mental status, Meningism, Papilledema, signs of sepsis (rash, shock), acute focal neurologic deficit, severe hypertension (e.g. systolic >220 mm Hg, or diastolic 120 mm Hg on consecutive readings) with any symptoms.

- Neuroimaging usually MRI should be done within hours or days in patients with the following- Focal neurologic deficit of subacute or uncertain onset, age > 50 years, weight loss, cancer, HIV infection, diplopia, change in an established headache pattern.

- ESR should be done if patients have visual symptoms, jaw or tongue claudication, tender or swollen temporal artery with reduced or absent pulses to look for temporal arteritis.

ABC approach to headache (evaluation + workup):

A — Assessment and immediate threats

Rapid severity check

- Obs/NEWS2, **GCS, capillary glucose**, pain score, vomiting, fever, BP (very high BP + neuro symptoms = emergency).

Immediate threats / red flags (urgent ED / same-day imaging or specialist pathway)

- **Subarachnoid haemorrhage (SAH): thunderclap** (max intensity in <1 min), "worst headache", collapse, meningism
- **Meningitis/encephalitis:** fever, neck stiffness, photophobia, rash, altered mental state, seizures
- **Stroke/ICH:** focal neurology, reduced consciousness, new seizures
- **Giant cell arteritis (age ≥50):** new headache + scalp tenderness, jaw claudication, visual symptoms
- **Acute glaucoma:** red painful eye, halos, reduced vision, nausea/vomiting
- **Cerebral venous sinus thrombosis (CVST):** headache + seizures/focal deficits/papilloedema; risk: pregnancy/postpartum, OCP, thrombophilia
- **Raised ICP / mass lesion:** morning headache, vomiting, papilloedema, worse with cough/strain, progressive pattern
- **Hypertensive emergency:** severe headache + end-organ signs (neuro, chest pain, AKI)

- **Carbon monoxide exposure:** headache with nausea/dizziness, multiple household members affected

Immediate actions if red flags

- ABCDE, analgesia/antiemetic, treat hypoglycaemia/hypoxia
- **Urgent neuro exam + fundoscopy** (papilloedema)
- **CT head (± CTA)** if SAH/ICH/stroke suspected; activate stroke pathway if appropriate
- If suspected **meningitis/encephalitis:** start **IV antibiotics** ± acyclovir per pathway (do not delay if septic or very unwell)
- **If suspected GCA:** take bloods (ESR/CRP, platelets) and **start high-dose steroids immediately**; urgent ophthalmology/rheum pathway
- If suspected **acute glaucoma:** urgent ophthalmology + IOP-lowering treatment per local protocol

B — Bedside assessment (focused history and exam)

Focused history

- **Onset/time course:** sudden vs gradual; first/worst; progressive; recurrent pattern
- **Character/location:** unilateral/bilateral, throbbing/pressure, occipital/temporal
- **Associated symptoms:**
  - **Migraine:** photophobia/phonophobia, nausea, aura, worse with activity
  - **Tension-type:** band-like tightness, no neuro deficit
  - **Cluster:** severe unilateral orbital/temporal + autonomic features (tearing, rhinorrhoea)

- Fever/rash/neck stiffness; visual symptoms; jaw claudication
- Neuro symptoms: weakness, speech change, seizures, confusion
- **Triggers/exposures:** exertion/sex (SAH), cough/strain (raised ICP), CO exposure, recent infection, trauma
- **Risk factors:** anticoagulation, pregnancy/postpartum/OCP (CVST), immunosuppression, cancer
- **Medication history:** analgesic overuse (MOH), nitrates, recent new meds

Focused exam

- **Vitals** (fever, severe HTN)
- **Neuro exam:** cranial nerves, limb power/sensation, coordination, gait
- **Meningism** (neck stiffness) if appropriate
- **Eye exam:** pupils, EOM, visual acuity/fields; **red painful eye**; fundoscopy for papilloedema
- **Temporal arteries** (tenderness, reduced pulse) if GCA suspected
- **Sinus/ENT** if facial pain/nasal discharge
- Consider **scalp tenderness/occipital neuralgia** features

C- Core investigations (workup)

If "primary headache" likely (migraine/tension/cluster) and no red flags

- Often **no investigations required**
- Consider diary + screen for medication overuse and secondary triggers

If red flags or atypical features

- **Bloods:** FBC, U&E, CRP ± ESR, glucose
- **CT head (non-contrast)** for suspected bleed/mass; **CTA** if aneurysm/SAH suspected or per pathway
- **Lumbar puncture:**
  - **If SAH suspected** with negative CT but ongoing suspicion (timing and local protocol dependent)
  - For suspected meningitis/encephalitis **after** imaging if indicated (e.g., focal neurology, immunosuppression, reduced GCS, papilloedema)
- **MRI brain if:**
  - Posterior fossa symptoms, suspected tumour, demyelination, chronic progressive headache, or CT non-diagnostic
- **MRV/CTV if CVST** suspected
- **ESR/CRP** + **platelets** urgently if **GCA** suspected (but **don't delay steroids**)
- **COHb** (venous blood gas) if carbon monoxide exposure suspected.

📑 **Mnemonic for Headache Red Flags: "SNOOP"**

- **S – Systemic symptoms (fever, weight loss) or Secondary risk factors (HIV, malignancy)**
- **N – Neurological signs or symptoms**
- **O – Onset sudden ("thunderclap")**
- **O – Older age (>50 years) at onset**
- **P – Progressive, positional, precipitated by exertion, or papilloedema**

Haematuria

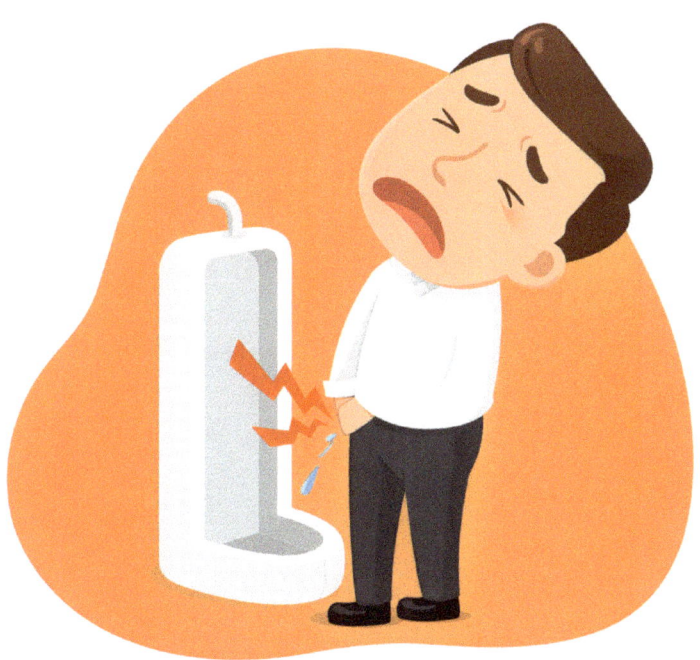

⚑ Red Flags: Haematuria

- ⚠ Painless Visible Haematuria (especially age >40 years)
- ⚠ Haematuria with Flank Pain or Palpable Mass
- ⚠ Haematuria with Clots
- ⚠ Haematuria with Proteinuria or Red Cell Casts
- ⚠ Haematuria with Systemic Symptoms (fever, night sweats, weight loss)
- ⚠ Haematuria after Recent Trauma
- ⚠ Haematuria with New-Onset Hypertension or Renal Impairment
- ⚠ Haematuria in Patients on Anticoagulants (Warfarin or DOACs)
- ⚠ Persistent Microscopic Haematuria (≥2 positive samples)
- ⚠ Age > 50
- ⚠ Hypertension & edema

∏ **Painless Visible Haematuria (especially age >40 years):**
- ❖ **Implications/Diagnoses:** This is a classic red flag for malignancy within the urinary tract. The most likely causes include bladder cancer (transitional cell carcinoma), renal cell carcinoma, and urothelial carcinoma of the renal pelvis or ureter. Less commonly, it may represent benign causes such as papillary necrosis or renal cyst rupture.
- ❖ **Investigations:** Urgent urological referral for flexible cystoscopy and CT urogram is essential. Include urine cytology, renal function tests, and FBC. If malignancy is

detected, staging scans (CT chest/abdomen/pelvis) may follow.

∏ Haematuria with Flank Pain or Palpable Mass:

- **Implications/Diagnoses:** Suggests a renal origin of bleeding. Differential diagnoses include renal cell carcinoma, renal or ureteric stones, hydronephrosis, and occasionally renal vein thrombosis. Flank mass plus haematuria is particularly concerning for renal malignancy.
- **Investigations:** Perform CT KUB (for stones) or CT urogram (for suspected tumour). Add urine microscopy for red cells and crystals, renal function, and ultrasound if CT is contraindicated.

∏ Haematuria with Dysuria, Urgency, or Frequency:

- **Implications/Diagnoses:** Usually caused by urinary tract infection (UTI), acute bacterial cystitis, or prostatitis, but recurrent or persistent symptoms can indicate bladder carcinoma or carcinoma in situ.
- **Investigations:** Perform urine dipstick, microscopy, and culture. If haematuria persists after infection treatment or recurs, proceed to cystoscopy and CT urogram. Repeat urine microscopy post-antibiotic therapy to confirm resolution.

∏ Haematuria with Clots:

- **Implications/Diagnoses:** Clot formation implies lower urinary tract bleeding. Common causes include bladder cancer, prostate cancer, urethral bleeding, benign prostatic hyperplasia (BPH), or traumatic catheterisation.
- **Investigations:** Conduct urgent cystoscopy to locate the bleeding source and CT urogram to assess upper tracts. In men over 50, check PSA and perform digital rectal examination (DRE).

∏ Haematuria with Proteinuria or Red Cell Casts:

- **Implications/Diagnoses:** This pattern suggests glomerular disease rather than a structural lesion. Diagnoses include IgA nephropathy, post-streptococcal glomerulonephritis, membranous GN, lupus nephritis, and ANCA-associated vasculitis.
- **Investigations:** Perform urine microscopy for dysmorphic RBCs and casts, urine protein: creatinine ratio (PCR), U&E/eGFR, and autoimmune screen (ANA, ANCA, complement levels). Renal biopsy may be indicated for diagnostic confirmation.

∏ Haematuria with Systemic Symptoms (fever, night sweats, weight loss):

- **Implications/Diagnoses:** These constitutional symptoms raise suspicion for malignancy (renal, bladder, or prostate cancer), renal tuberculosis, or systemic vasculitis (e.g. granulomatosis with polyangiitis).
- **Investigations:**: Arrange CT urogram, urine for AFB and mycobacterial culture, autoimmune profile, ESR/CRP, and FBC. Consider chest X-ray if TB or vasculitis is suspected.

∏ Haematuria after Recent Trauma:

- **Implications/Diagnoses:** Indicative of renal, ureteric, or bladder injury due to blunt or penetrating trauma. Possible injuries include renal laceration, renal pedicle injury, or bladder rupture.
- **Investigations:** Order CT abdomen/pelvis with contrast (trauma protocol) to assess for renal or vascular damage. If bladder injury suspected, perform a retrograde cystogram.

∏ Haematuria with New-Onset Hypertension or Renal Impairment:

- ❖ **Implications/Diagnoses:** Suggests glomerulonephritis, vasculitis, or malignant hypertension causing renal vascular injury. Common causes include rapidly progressive GN, Goodpasture's syndrome, and polyarteritis nodosa.
- ❖ **Investigations:** Check U&E/eGFR, urine microscopy for RBC casts, autoimmune and vasculitis screen, and renal ultrasound for kidney size and echogenicity.

∏ Haematuria in Patients on Anticoagulants (Warfarin or DOACs):

- ❖ **Implications/Diagnoses:** Though anticoagulation can exacerbate bleeding, it may reveal an underlying pathology such as bladder cancer, renal tumour, or urothelial carcinoma.
- ❖ **Investigations:** Check INR (for warfarin) or drug level (for DOACs). If haematuria persists after correcting anticoagulation, perform cystoscopy and CT urogram. Always exclude malignancy before attributing the bleeding to medication.

∏ Persistent Microscopic Haematuria (≥2 positive samples):

- ❖ **Implications/Diagnoses:** Persistent microscopic haematuria may indicate early bladder or renal cancer, glomerulonephritis, or urolithiasis. Even in asymptomatic patients, this should not be ignored.
- ❖ **Investigations:** Repeat urine microscopy and perform renal function tests and autoimmune screen. Arrange renal ultrasound or CT urogram, and cystoscopy for patients over 40 or with risk factors such as smoking or chemical exposure.

∏ Age > 50 years:

- ❖ **Implications/Diagnoses:** Strongly suggests urological malignancy, particularly transitional cell carcinoma of the bladder or renal cell carcinoma. Could also indicate benign prostatic hyperplasia (BPH) causing obstruction and bleeding. Less likely but possible: renal or ureteric calculi in older adults.

- ❖ **Investigations:** Urinalysis and microscopy – to confirm haematuria, look for dysmorphic RBCs or casts, Urine cytology – for malignant cells, CT urogram (CT IVP) – first-line imaging for upper urinary tract malignancy, Cystoscopy – gold standard to evaluate the bladder for tumour or bleeding source, PSA (in men) and digital rectal exam – to assess for prostate pathology.

∏ Hypertension and Edema:

- ❖ **Implications/Diagnoses:** Suggests a glomerular (renal parenchymal) cause rather than urological, Glomerulonephritis (e.g. IgA nephropathy, post-streptococcal GN, lupus nephritis), Nephritic syndrome pattern (haematuria, hypertension, reduced renal function, mild proteinuria), May also indicate chronic kidney disease (CKD) with secondary hypertension and fluid retention.

- ❖ **Investigations:** Urinalysis – red cell casts and proteinuria suggest glomerular origin, Urine protein: creatinine ratio (PCR) or albumin: creatinine ratio (ACR). Renal function tests (U&E, eGFR) – assess kidney impairment. Renal ultrasound – to evaluate kidney size and chronic changes. Autoimmune screen – ANA, ANCA, complement levels, anti-GBM if GN suspected. Renal biopsy – definitive for glomerulonephritis diagnosis if indicated.

🗝️ Key Points:

- Visible haematuria is malignancy until proven otherwise.
- Always exclude infection first and repeat urinalysis after treatment.
- Combine upper tract imaging and cystoscopy for complete evaluation.
- Persistent microscopic haematuria or haematuria with abnormal renal parameters requires nephrology input.
- Risk of serious disease increases with aging and with duration and degree of haematuria.
- The most common specific causes differ somewhat by age, but overall the most common are:- UTI, Prostatitis, Urinary calculi, cancer and prostate disease are a more of a concern in patients > 50, although younger patients with risk factors may occasionally develop cancer. Glomerular disease can be a cause in all ages.

ABC approach to haematuria (evaluation + workup):

A — Assessment and immediate threats

Rapid severity check

- Obs/NEWS2, pain score, urine output, degree of bleeding (**clots?**), haemodynamic stability.

Immediate threats / red flags (urgent same-day / ED / urology)

- **Clot retention / acute urinary retention:** suprapubic pain/distension, inability to void
- **Haemodynamic instability** or ongoing heavy bleeding
- **Obstructed infected system:** fever/rigors + flank pain + hydronephrosis/AKI risk (stone + infection) → urgent urology

- **Severe flank pain** suggestive of **stone** (especially with fever, solitary kidney, or AKI)
- **Trauma** (renal injury) or recent urological instrumentation
- **Anticoagulated** patient with significant bleeding
- **Pregnancy** (urgent assessment; broaden differential)

Immediate actions if red flags

- IV access, analgesia, fluids if needed
- **Urinalysis**; send **MSU culture**
- **Bloods:** FBC, U&E/creatinine, CRP (if infection), coagulation if on anticoagulants/heavy bleed
- If clot retention: **3-way catheter + bladder irrigation** (per local policy) and urgent urology review
- If sepsis/obstruction suspected: antibiotics + **urgent imaging** and urology

B — Bedside assessment (focused history and exam)

Focused history

- **Type:** visible (macroscopic) vs non-visible (microscopic); first episode or recurrent
- **Painful vs painless**
  - **Painless visible haematuria** → malignancy until proven otherwise
  - Pain + LUTS → UTI/stone more likely
- **Associated urinary symptoms:** dysuria, frequency, urgency, nocturia, hesitancy, poor stream
- **Flank pain/colic**, fever/rigors (pyelo/stone)
- **Clots:** suggest lower tract source; ask about retention

- **Timing:** initial/terminal/total haematuria (may suggest urethral/prostatic vs bladder/upper tract)
- **Recent exercise**, menstruation/contamination, recent infection
- **Risk factors for malignancy:** age, **smoking**, occupational exposures (dyes/rubber), pelvic radiotherapy, cyclophosphamide, chronic catheter
- **PMH:** stones, recurrent UTIs, BPH, known renal disease (proteinuria), bleeding disorders
- **Meds:** anticoagulants/antiplatelets (do not assume they are the sole cause)

Focused exam
- Vitals (fever, shock)
- Abdomen: suprapubic distension (retention), tenderness
- **CVA tenderness** (upper tract)
- External genital exam if indicated
- **DRE** in men if LUTS/prostate pathology suspected
- Look for systemic signs of renal disease (oedema, hypertension, rash/arthralgia)

C- Core investigations (workup)

Initial tests (most patients)
- **Urine dip** (blood, protein, nitrites/leukocytes)
- **Urine microscopy/culture** (especially if symptomatic or dip suggests infection)
- **FBC** (anaemia), **U&E/creatinine** (renal function)
- Consider **ACR/PCR** if proteinuria (suggests glomerular cause)

Imaging (choose based on risk and presentation)

- **Suspected stone/renal colic: CT KUB** (non-pregnant) or **renal US** (pregnancy)
- **High-risk haematuria / visible haematuria:** upper tract imaging (often **CT urogram** per pathway; US if CT not suitable)

Cancer evaluation (key)

- **Visible (macroscopic) haematuria** typically needs **urgent urology assessment** with:
    - **Cystoscopy** (lower tract)
    - **Upper tract imaging** (CT urogram or equivalent pathway)

When to think glomerular

- Haematuria + **proteinuria**, hypertension, oedema, AKI, or dysmorphic RBCs/casts
    - Add: ACR/PCR, serum albumin, complements/autoimmune tests **if clinically indicated**
    - Consider nephrology referral

Other

- **Pregnancy test** where relevant
- PSA is **not** a haematuria test (only if prostate symptoms/assessment indicated)

Haematuria decision bullets (visible vs dip-only; painful vs painless)

1) Visible haematuria (macroscopic)
- **Painless visible haematuria**
    - **Assume malignancy until proven otherwise** (bladder/renal/upper tract).
    - **Urgent urology referral for cystoscopy + upper tract imaging** (often CT urogram per local pathway).
- **Painful visible haematuria**
    - Think **UTI**, **stone**, prostatitis, (less commonly) tumour with clots/irritation.
    - **If fever/rigors/flank pain or AKI/solitary kidney → urgent imaging + urology** (obstructed infected system risk).
    - If classic renal colic and stable → analgesia + **CT KUB** (or renal USS if pregnant) + urine culture if infection possible.
- **Visible haematuria with clots / retention**
    - **Emergency urology** (clot retention): 3-way catheter + irrigation per policy.

2) Dip-only haematuria (non-visible / microscopic)
- **Painful dip-only haematuria**
    - Often **UTI** or **stone**.
    - Do **urine culture**, treat if UTI; image if colicky flank pain or recurrent.
- **Painless dip-only haematuria**
    - Repeat to confirm (exclude contamination/exercise/menstruation).

- Check for **proteinuria (ACR/PCR)**, BP, creatinine:
  - **Proteinuria/HTN/AKI/oedema → glomerular cause likely → nephrology pathway**
  - **No proteinuria + persistent haematuria or risk factors (age, smoking) → urology pathway** per local guideline.

Quick rule of thumb

- **Visible + painless = cancer pathway**
- **Pain + fever/rigors or obstruction signs = emergency (infected obstruction)**
- **Dip-only + proteinuria/AKI/HTN = nephrology (glomerular)**
- **Dip-only + no renal features but persistent/risk factors = urology**

📃 Mnemonic Red Flags for Haematuria: **BLOOD ALERT**

B – Bleeding that is painless and visible

→ Suggests bladder or renal malignancy (e.g. transitional cell carcinoma, renal cell carcinoma).

L – Lump or flank pain

→ May indicate a renal mass (RCC) or renal/ureteric calculi.

O – Old age (>40 years)

→ Increases suspicion of urothelial or renal cancer — malignancy until proven otherwise.

O – On anticoagulants but haematuria persists

→ May unmask an underlying tumour; not to be dismissed as a drug effect alone.

D – Dysuria, frequency, or urgency that persists after antibiotics

→ Could indicate bladder carcinoma or carcinoma in situ.

A – Associated proteinuria or red cell casts

→ Points to glomerular disease such as IgA nephropathy, GN, or vasculitis.

L – Loss of weight, fever, or night sweats

→ Suggests malignancy, renal tuberculosis, or systemic vasculitis.

E – Elevated blood pressure or renal impairment

→ Consistent with glomerulonephritis, vasculitis, or malignant hypertension.

R – Recent trauma

→ Indicates possible renal or bladder injury.

T – Two or more positive urine microscopy samples (persistent microscopic haematuria)

→ May signify early renal or urological malignancy or glomerular disease.

🧠 Quick Recall Phrase for Mnemonic:

"When you see BLOOD, be on ALERT — every drop could signal danger."

Hemoptysis

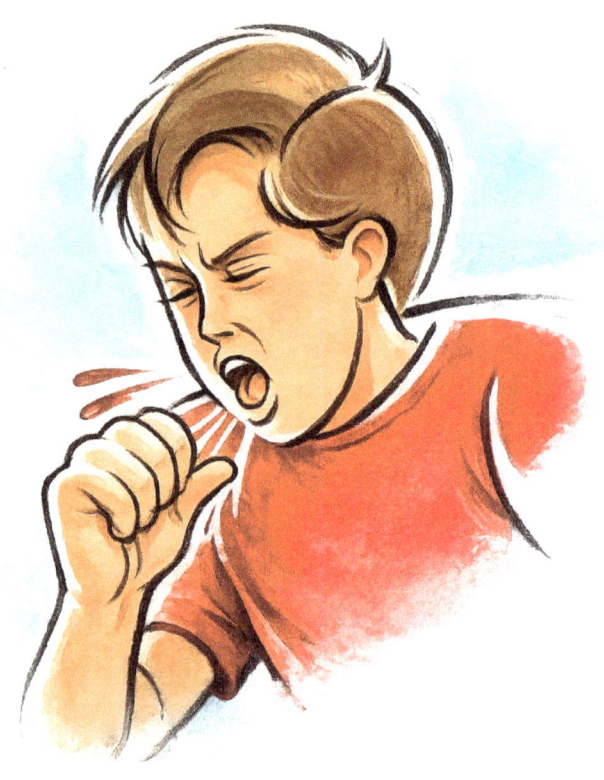

▶ Red Flags: Hemoptysis

- ⚠ Massive haemoptysis (>150 mL in 24 hours or life-threatening bleeding)
- ⚠ Age >40 years, smoker, or unexplained haemoptysis
- ⚠ Recurrent or persistent haemoptysis
- ⚠ Systemic symptoms (fever, weight loss, night sweats, malaise)
- ⚠ Haemoptysis with haematuria or renal impairment
- ⚠ History of tuberculosis or travel to endemic areas
- ⚠ Dyspnoea, pleuritic chest pain, haemoptysis, tachycardia
- ⚠ Immunocompromised state (HIV, chemotherapy, transplant)
- ⚠ Associated cardiac findings (orthopnoea, PND, leg swelling)
- ⚠ Anticoagulant or bleeding tendency

∏ **Massive haemoptysis (>150 mL in 24 hours or life-threatening bleeding):**

- ❖ **Implications/Diagnoses:** Pulmonary artery erosion or bronchial artery rupture, Bronchiectasis with vessel erosion, Cavitary tuberculosis, Pulmonary malignancy, Pulmonary embolism with infarction.
- ❖ **Investigations:** Urgent ABC assessment, oxygen saturation, airway protection, Chest X-ray → look for consolidation, cavitation, mass, CT pulmonary angiography (CTPA) → identify source and vascular lesion, Bronchoscopy (urgent)

→ localise site and control bleeding, Group and crossmatch, coagulation screen

∏ Age >40 years, smoker, or unexplained haemoptysis:
- **Implications/Diagnoses:** Bronchogenic carcinoma until proven otherwise, Chronic bronchitis or COPD with superimposed malignancy
- **Investigations:** Chest X-ray → if normal, proceed further, CT thorax (high-resolution or contrast) → detect small or central lesions, Bronchoscopy → direct visualisation and biopsy, Sputum cytology.

∏ Recurrent or persistent haemoptysis:
- **Implications/Diagnoses:** Bronchiectasis, chronic infection, or malignancy, Tuberculosis, aspergilloma, or vasculitis (GPA, Goodpasture's)
- **Investigations:** HRCT thorax → evaluate for bronchiectasis, cavitation, AFB sputum and TB PCR, ANCA and anti-GBM antibodies, Bronchoscopy for local pathology.

∏ Systemic symptoms (fever, weight loss, night sweats, malaise):
- **Implications/Diagnoses:** Tuberculosis, Lung abscess, Malignancy, Autoimmune vasculitis.
- **Investigations:** CXR/CT chest for cavitation or infiltrates, Sputum AFB × 3, culture, ESR/CRP, autoimmune screen (ANCA), HIV test if risk factors present.

∏ Haemoptysis with haematuria or renal impairment:
- **Implications/Diagnoses:** Goodpasture's syndrome, Granulomatosis with polyangiitis (Wegener's), Pulmonary–renal vasculitis syndromes.
- **Investigations:** Urinalysis → blood, protein, casts, Renal function (U&E, creatinine), Autoimmune screen → ANCA,

anti-GBM, ANA, CXR → diffuse alveolar infiltrates, CT chest ± bronchoscopy.

∏ History of tuberculosis or travel to endemic areas:

- ❖ **Implications/Diagnoses:** Active or reactivation TB, Post-TB bronchiectasis or aspergilloma
- ❖ **Investigations:** Sputum AFB × 3 and TB culture → cavitation, apical fibrosis, CT chest for structural changes, Serum Aspergillus IgG if fungal ball suspected.

∏ Dyspnoea, pleuritic chest pain, haemoptysis, tachycardia:

- ❖ **Implications/Diagnoses:** Pulmonary embolism (PE with infarction)
- ❖ **Investigations:** D-dimer (if low pretest probability), CT pulmonary angiogram (CTPA), ABG → hypoxia, respiratory alkalosis, ECG → sinus tachycardia, right heart strain pattern.

∏ Immunocompromised state (HIV, chemotherapy, transplant):

- ❖ **Implications/Diagnoses:** Invasive aspergillosis, Pneumocystis jirovecii pneumonia (PJP), Cytomegalovirus infection
- ❖ **Investigations:** CT chest (halo sign, nodules), BAL for fungal culture/PCR, HIV testing, CD4 count, Galactomannan antigen or β-D-glucan assay.

∏ Associated cardiac findings (orthopnoea, PND, leg swelling):

- ❖ **Implications/Diagnoses:** Mitral stenosis (elevated pulmonary venous pressure), Left ventricular failure.
- ❖ **Investigations:** Echocardiogram → assess mitral valve and LV function, BNP, CXR → pulmonary oedema, cardiomegaly.

∏ Anticoagulant or bleeding tendency:

- ❖ **Implications/Diagnoses:** Over-anticoagulation (warfarin, DOAC), Thrombocytopenia, coagulopathy.

- **Investigations:** INR, PT, aPTT, platelet count, Medication review, CXR/CT to exclude concomitant pathology.

🗝 Key points:

- Massive haemoptysis → main cause of death is asphyxia, not exsanguination
- Bronchial artery embolization = first-line definitive therapy for massive haemoptysis
- CT angiography helps localize bleeding and guide embolization
- Always rule out malignancy in recurrent or older patients

ABC approach to haemoptysis (evaluation + workup):

A — Assessment and immediate threats

1) Confirm it's haemoptysis (not haematemesis/pseudohaemoptysis)

- **Haemoptysis:** coughing blood, frothy, mixed with sputum
- **Haematemesis:** vomiting blood, "coffee grounds", GI symptoms
- **Pseudohaemoptysis:** bleeding from nose/oropharynx

2) Rapid severity check

- Obs/NEWS2: **SpO_2, RR, HR, BP,** work of breathing
- Estimate volume + rate (even rough): **ongoing bleeding?** clots?
- Look for **respiratory failure or shock**

3) Immediate threats / red flags (treat as emergency)

- **Massive / life-threatening haemoptysis** (any of):
  - Airway compromise, hypoxia, inability to clear blood
  - Haemodynamic instability
  - Rapid ongoing bleeding / large volume
- **Suspected pulmonary embolism** (pleuritic pain, tachycardia, hypoxia, DVT signs)
- **TB** risk (fever, night sweats, weight loss, exposure) or severe pneumonia/sepsis
- **Known lung cancer**, significant smoking history, or recurrent/unexplained haemoptysis
- **Anticoagulation/bleeding diathesis**

Immediate actions (first minutes)

- Call for help early (senior/anaesthetics/ICU; respiratory/interventional radiology if severe)
- High-flow O_2 if needed; IV access x2; bloods + crossmatch
- **Position bleeding lung down** (if known) to protect the other lung
- Stop/reverse anticoagulants **if major bleeding** per local pathway
- If unstable: prepare for **airway control** (intubation with large-bore tube) and urgent definitive therapy (bronchoscopy/embolisation)

B — Bedside assessment (focused history and exam)

Focused history

- **Volume & pattern:** streaks vs cups; single episode vs recurrent; clots

- **Symptoms:** fever, purulent sputum, pleuritic pain, dyspnoea, wheeze, weight loss, night sweats
- **Risk factors / PMH:**
  - **Bronchiectasis**, COPD, TB/previous TB, pneumonia
  - Malignancy, autoimmune disease (vasculitis), heart disease (mitral stenosis)
  - VTE risk (recent surgery/immobility, cancer, OCP/pregnancy)
- **Drugs: anticoagulants/antiplatelets**, NSAIDs; cocaine/inhaled irritants
- **Bleeding source check:** epistaxis, gum bleeding, vomiting blood

Focused exam

- Vitals + respiratory distress
- ENT/oropharynx (look for source)
- Chest: crackles/focal signs, wheeze, reduced breath sounds
- CVS: murmurs (e.g., mitral stenosis), signs of HF
- Peripheral: DVT signs, petechiae/purpura (vasculitis), cachexia

C- Core investigations (workup)

Core tests for most patients.

- **CXR** (first-line)
- **Bloods:** FBC, U&E, LFT**, CRP,** coagulation profile (INR/PT/aPTT)
- **Group & save (crossmatch if moderate/severe)**
- **Sputum** culture if productive/infective features

- **ECG** ± troponin if chest pain/strain; ABG/VBG if hypoxic or severe

Targeted tests (based on suspicion)
- **CT chest with contrast / CT pulmonary angiography:**
  - If **moderate–severe haemoptysis**, abnormal CXR, high cancer risk, or unclear source
  - If **PE** suspected → **CTPA** per pathway
- **Bronchoscopy:**
  - If ongoing bleeding, need airway protection/localisation, or suspicion of endobronchial lesion
- **TB testing (if r**isk/symptoms): sputum AFB x3 ± NAAT; isolate if high suspicion
- **Autoimmune/renal** workup if vasculitis suspected (e.g., haemoptysis + AKI/proteinuria/purpura): urinalysis, ACR, creatinine trend ± ANCA/anti-GBM/complements (guided by clinical picture)
- **Echocardiography** if mitral stenosis/pulmonary venous hypertension suspected

When to escalate urgently
- Any **life-threatening haemoptysis** → ICU/anaesthetics + urgent CT/bronchoscopy ± **bronchial artery embolisatio**n (definitive in many cases) depending on local service.

Haemoptysis "streaks vs moderate vs massive" — bullet ladder

1) Streaks / small-volume (non–life-threatening)
- Typical: blood-streaked sputum or a few teaspoons, **no hypoxia**, haemodynamically stable, bleeding stopped.

- **Do now**
  - Obs + confirm source (ENT/GI vs lung)
  - **CXR, FBC + coag**, CRP ± sputum culture if productive
- **Likely causes:** acute bronchitis, mild infection, asthma/COPD flare, bronchiectasis.
- **Discharge may be reasonable if ALL true**
  - Stable obs, **SpO$_2$ normal**, no ongoing bleed
  - No red flags (weight loss, recurrent episodes, TB risk, cancer risk)
  - Clear safety-net + follow-up arranged
- **Arrange follow-up / further tests if**
  - Smoker/age risk, recurrent haemoptysis, abnormal CXR → **CT chest** ± respiratory referral

2) Moderate haemoptysis (needs admission/urgent imaging)

Typical: more than streaks (e.g., mouthfuls), recurrent over hours–days, or risk factors; may be mild hypoxia but stable BP.

- **Do now**
  - Admit, oxygen as needed, IV access
  - **CXR + bloods** (FBC, U&E, CRP, coag) + group & save
  - Treat likely infection if clinically indicated
- **Choose imaging**
  - **CT chest with contrast** to localise source and look for malignancy/bronchiectasis
  - **CTPA** if PE suspected (pleuritic pain, tachycardia, hypoxia, DVT signs)

- **Escalate**
  - Early respiratory input; consider bronchoscopy if persistent bleeding or suspected endobronchial lesion

3) Massive / life-threatening haemoptysis (resus + definitive control)

Practical definition: **any volume causing** airway compromise, hypoxia, inability to clear blood, or haemodynamic instability (volume cut-offs vary).

- **Immediate actions**
  - Call **anaesthetics/ICU + senior respiratory**; activate major haemorrhage if needed
  - High-flow O_2; **2 large-bore IVs**; crossmatch; correct coagulopathy
  - **Position bleeding side down** (if known) to protect the other lung
  - Prepare for **airway control** (intubation with large-bore tube)
- **Definitive localisation/control (often in parallel)**
  - **CT angiography (chest)** if stable enough to transfer → guides embolisation
  - **Urgent bronchoscopy** if unstable, to suction/localise/temporise
  - **Bronchial artery embolisation** is commonly definitive when available
  - Surgery if embolisation fails or specific surgical lesion

Quick "who gets what" (one-liners)

- **Stable + streaks + normal CXR** → basic labs ± treat infection; outpatient follow-up if no risk factors.

- **Moderate/recurrent OR abnormal CXR OR cancer/TB risk → CT chest (± CTPA)** + admit.
- **Any airway compromise/hypoxia/instability → massive pathway** (ICU/anaesthetics) + bronchoscopy/CTA → embolisation.

Mnemonic for Red Flags in Haemoptysis – "HAEMOPTYSIS"

H	Haemoptysis >150 mL/24 hr	Massive bleed (life-threatening)
A	Age >40, smoker	Bronchogenic carcinoma
E	Endemic area / past TB	Tuberculosis / aspergilloma
M	Multiple episodes	Bronchiectasis / malignancy
O	Other bleeding (haematuria)	Vasculitis / Goodpasture's
P	Pleuritic pain, dyspnoea	Pulmonary embolism
T	Temperature, weight loss	TB / malignancy
Y	Yellow (immunosuppressed)	Opportunistic infection
S	Smoker with chronic cough	Carcinoma / chronic bronchitis
I	INR high / on anticoagulants	Coagulopathy
S	Signs of heart failure	Mitral stenosis / LV failure

Jaundice

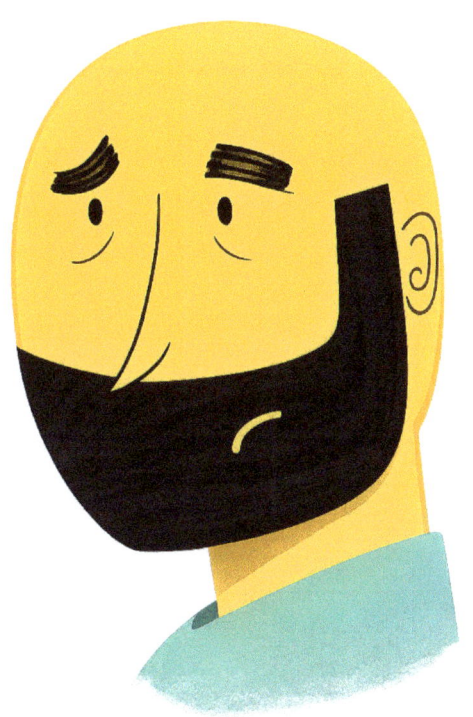

🚩 Red Flags: Jaundice

- ⚠ **Painless progressive jaundice (especially in an older patient)**
- ⚠ **Jaundice with fever and right upper quadrant pain (Charcot's triad)**
- ⚠ **Acute jaundice with encephalopathy or coagulopathy**
- ⚠ **Jaundice with severe abdominal pain radiating to back**
- ⚠ **Jaundice with anaemia, dark urine, and splenomegaly**
- ⚠ **Jaundice with weight loss, anorexia, or pruritus**
- ⚠ **Jaundice with confusion, asterixis, and fetor hepaticus**
- ⚠ **Jaundice with ascites, spider naevi, or variceal bleeding**
- ⚠ **Jaundice after recent drug exposure (antibiotics, paracetamol, anti-TB drugs, statins)**
- ⚠ **Jaundice in a neonate or pregnancy**

∏ Painless progressive jaundice (especially in an older patient):

- ❖ **Implications / Diagnoses:** Pancreatic head carcinoma, Cholangiocarcinoma, Ampullary carcinoma, Malignant biliary obstruction.
- ❖ **Investigations:** LFTs → Cholestatic pattern (↑ALP, ↑GGT, mild ↑ALT/AST), Ultrasound abdomen → Bile duct dilatation ("double duct sign"), CT abdomen / MRI with MRCP → Define level and cause of obstruction, Endoscopic ultrasound (EUS) or ERCP for tissue diagnosis / stenting, CA 19-9 tumour marker.

∏ Jaundice with fever and right upper quadrant pain (Charcot's triad):

- **Implications / Diagnoses:** Ascending cholangitis, May progress to sepsis or hepatic abscess.
- **Investigations:** Blood cultures, LFTs → Marked cholestasis, Ultrasound or MRCP → Common bile duct stones / obstruction, CBC → Leucocytosis, Urgent ERCP → Diagnostic and therapeutic.

∏ Acute jaundice with encephalopathy or coagulopathy:

- **Implications / Diagnoses:** Acute liver failure (fulminant hepatitis, paracetamol toxicity, viral, autoimmune), Massive hepatic necrosis
- **Investigations:** LFTs → Very high ALT/AST, ↑bilirubin, prolonged INR, Prothrombin time / INR → prognostic marker, Ammonia level → hepatic encephalopathy, Serum paracetamol, viral hepatitis panel, autoimmune screen, Urgent transfer to liver unit.

∏ Jaundice with severe abdominal pain radiating to back:

- **Implications / Diagnoses:** Gallstone pancreatitis, Pancreatic head mass.
- **Investigations:** Serum amylase / lipase, Ultrasound / CT abdomen → gallstones, pancreatic inflammation or mass, LFTs → Obstructive pattern, MRCP / ERCP if biliary obstruction suspected.

∏ Jaundice with anaemia, dark urine, and splenomegaly:

- **Implications / Diagnoses:** Haemolytic jaundice, Possible causes: autoimmune haemolysis, malaria, hereditary spherocytosis, G6PD deficiency

- ❖ **Investigations:** Peripheral blood film (spherocytes, schistocytes), Reticulocyte count → raised, LDH, haptoglobin (↑LDH, ↓haptoglobin), Direct antiglobulin (Coombs) test, Bilirubin pattern → unconjugated predominance.

∏ Jaundice with weight loss, anorexia, or pruritus:
- ❖ **Implications / Diagnoses:** Malignant obstructive jaundice (cholangiocarcinoma, pancreatic cancer), Primary biliary cholangitis (PBC) or Primary sclerosing cholangitis (PSC)
- ❖ **Investigations:** LFTs → Cholestatic pattern, Ultrasound / MRCP → ductal dilatation or beading, AMA / ANA / p-ANCA, CA 19-9, CEA for malignancy screening.

∏ Jaundice with confusion, asterixis, and fetor hepaticus:
- ❖ **Implications / Diagnoses:** Hepatic encephalopathy secondary to chronic liver disease or acute liver failure
- ❖ **Investigations:** Ammonia level, LFTs, INR, ABG, Ultrasound / Doppler → portal hypertension, shunts, Exclude precipitating factors (infection, bleed, constipation, sedatives).

∏ Jaundice with ascites, spider naevi, or variceal bleeding:
- ❖ **Implications / Diagnoses:** Decompensated cirrhosis (alcoholic, viral, NASH, autoimmune, etc.).
- ❖ **Investigations:** LFTs → deranged synthetic function, Ultrasound abdomen → cirrhotic liver, portal hypertension, Ascitic fluid analysis → SAAG, culture, cytology, Endoscopy → oesophageal varices.

∏ Jaundice after recent drug exposure (antibiotics, paracetamol, anti-TB drugs, statins):
- ❖ **Implications / Diagnoses:** Drug-induced liver injury (DILI) — hepatocellular, cholestatic, or mixed pattern
- ❖ **Investigations:** LFTs → pattern depending on type of injury,

Drug history and withdrawal, Autoimmune / viral screen to exclude other causes, Liver biopsy if uncertain.

∏ Jaundice in pregnancy:

- ❖ **Implications / Diagnoses:** Pregnancy-. acute fatty liver, HELLP syndrome, intrahepatic cholestasis
- ❖ **Investigations:** Pregnancy-specific labs: LFTs, coagulation, platelet count, Ultrasound / Doppler.

🗝 Key points:

- In an otherwise young and health acute jaundice suggests acute viral hepatitis.
- In elderly patients with painless jaundice with weight loss, an abdominal mass suggests biliary obstruction caused by cancer.
- Aminotransferase (ALT) of > 500 U/L and alkaline phosphatase elevation (ALP) < 3 times normal suggests hepatocellular dysfunction.
- ALT levels of < 200U/L and ALP >3 times normal suggest cholestasis.
- Altered mental state and coagulopathy indicates significant hepatic dysfunction.
- **Dark urine + pale stool** → conjugated bilirubin → *obstructive pattern*.
- **Isolated bilirubin rise** with normal enzymes → *Gilbert's syndrome* (benign)
- **Painless jaundice + palpable gallbladder (Courvoisier sign)** → likely *malignancy*
- Always check **drug and alcohol history** in any jaundiced patient
- "3 H's Rule"-

- **H**aemolytic → pre-hepatic
  Hepatocellular → intra-hepatic
  Hepatobiliary → post-hepatic

ABC approach to jaundice (evaluation + workup):

A — Assessment and immediate threats

Rapid severity check

- Obs/NEWS2, mental state (encephalopathy), pain, hydration, bleeding/bruising, glucose.

Immediate threats / red flags (urgent same-day / ED / specialist)

- **Ascending cholangitis** (biliary sepsis): **fever + RUQ pain + jaundice** (± hypotension/confusion)
- **Acute liver failure:** jaundice + **INR raised/bleeding** ± encephalopathy, hypoglycaemia
- **Severe hepatitis/toxin** (e.g., paracetamol): systemic illness, vomiting, marked transaminitis
- **Obstructed system** (stone/stricture/malignancy) with sepsis or worsening pain
- **GI bleed** / significant coagulopathy
- **Severe haemolysis** (anaemia, cardiovascular compromise)

Immediate actions if red flags

- IV access, fluids, analgesia/antiemetic; treat hypoglycaemia
- **Bloods urgently:** FBC, U&E, LFTs, **INR/PT**, albumin, CRP, glucose
- **Blood cultures** if febrile; start **IV antibiotics** if cholangitis suspected
- Early **urgent ultrasound** (biliary obstruction) and specialist referral

- If suspected acute liver failure/paracetamol: follow **toxicology/liver unit** pathway; consider NAC per protocol

B — Bedside assessment (focused history and exam)

Focused history (localize pattern)

- **Onset & course:** sudden vs progressive; pale stools/dark urine; pruritus
- **Pain:** RUQ colic (stones), constant RUQ (cholecystitis/cholangitis), painless jaundice (malignancy more likely)
- **Systemic:** fever/rigors, weight loss, night sweats, anorexia
- **Hepatitis risks:** alcohol binge/chronic use, viral exposure (travel, IVDU, sex, tattoos), recent illness, sick contacts
- **Drug/toxin:** paracetamol (dose/time), antibiotics (e.g., co-amoxiclav), statins, herbals, anabolic steroids
- **Haemolysis clues:** fatigue, dark urine without pale stools, recent infection/drugs, known haemoglobinopathy
- **PMH:** gallstones, pancreatitis, liver disease/cirrhosis, cancer, transfusions
- **Pregnancy** (cholestasis/HELLP), family history

Focused exam

- General: jaundice, scratch marks, cachexia
- Vitals: fever, hypotension
- Abdomen: RUQ tenderness, hepatomegaly, palpable gallbladder, masses, ascites
- Stigmata of chronic liver disease: spider naevi, palmar erythema, gynaecomastia, splenomegaly
- Neuro: asterixis, confusion (encephalopathy)
- Signs of bleeding: bruising, petechiae

C- Core investigations (workup)

Core labs (first line for most)

- **LFTs** (bilirubin, ALT/AST, ALP, GGT), **albumin**
- **Coagulation: INR/PT**
- **FBC** (anaemia, platelets), **U&E/creatinine**
- **CRP** (infection), **glucose**

Interpret pattern + next tests.

1) Cholestatic pattern (ALP/GGT >> ALT/AST) ± pale stools/dark urine/pruritus

- **Ultrasound RUQ (first line)** to look for biliary dilatation/gallstones
- If dilated ducts or strong suspicion despite normal US:
  - **MRCP** (diagnostic) ± **EUS**
  - **ERCP** if **therapeutic** needed (stone/stricture) or cholangitis
- Add: **CA 19-9** only in specialist pathway (not diagnostic alone)

2) Hepatocellular pattern (ALT/AST >> ALP)

- **Viral hepatitis screen** (HAV IgM, HBsAg/anti-HBc IgM, HCV Ab/Ag ± PCR depending on pathway)
- **Paracetamol level** if any possibility (even if history unclear)
- Consider autoimmune/metabolic if unexplained or persistent: ANA/SMA/IgG, ferritin/transferrin saturation, ceruloplasmin (young), A1AT (selected)

3) Haemolytic / pre-hepatic pattern (isolated bilirubin rise, often unconjugated)

- **Haemolysis screen:** retics, LDH, haptoglobin, blood film, DAT
- Check for anaemia and triggers (drugs, infection)

Imaging and escalation

- **CT abdomen/pancreas** if painless progressive jaundice, weight loss, mass suspected, or US suggests malignancy
- **Urgent referral:**
  - Suspected **cholangitis** → urgent biliary decompression pathway
  - **INR raised/encephalopathy** → acute liver failure/liver unit pathway

📖 Mnemonic for Red Flags in Jaundice — "JAUNDICED"

Letter Red Flag	Likely Cause
J Jaundice painless & progressive	Pancreatic / biliary cancer
A Altered sensorium / coagulopathy	Acute liver failure
U Upper abdominal pain & fever	Ascending cholangitis
N New-onset with severe pain	Gallstone pancreatitis
D Dark urine + anaemia + splenomegaly	Haemolysis
I Itching & weight loss	Cholestatic malignancy / PBC
C Confusion / coma	Hepatic encephalopathy
E Exposure to hepatotoxic drugs	DILI
D Decompensation (ascites, varices)	Cirrhosis

Joint Pains

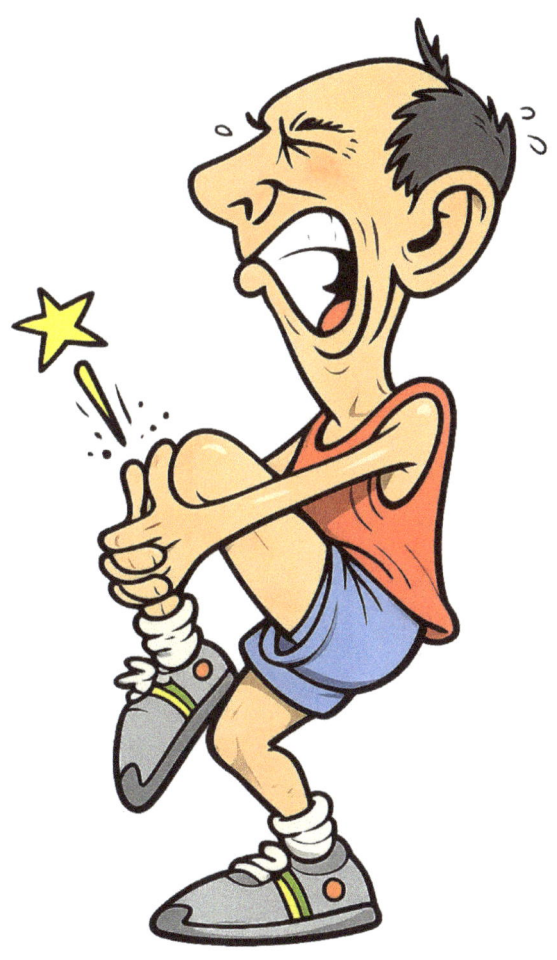

Red Flags: Joint pain & swelling

- Fever, rigors, or systemic toxicity
- Sudden onset of severe monoarthritis
- Hot, red, swollen joint (especially single large joint)
- Rapidly progressive joint destruction or deformity
- Weight loss, night sweats, or constitutional symptoms
- Polyarthritis with rash, mucosal ulcers, or serositis
- Back pain, stiffness, or enthesitis with peripheral arthritis
- Multiple joint involvement with early morning stiffness > 30 mins
- History of recent infection (especially GI/GU) preceding arthritis
- Hemarthrosis or easy bruising
- Pain out of proportion, severe tenderness, or inability to move joint
- Associated neuropathy, sensory loss, or painless swelling

∏ Fever, rigors, or systemic toxicity:
- **Implications / Diagnoses:** Suggests septic arthritis, osteomyelitis, or infective endocarditis–associated arthritis. Can also indicate inflammatory arthritis flare with infection.
- **Investigations:** Urgent joint aspiration → Gram stain, culture, WCC, crystals., Blood cultures, FBC, CRP/ESR, X-ray / Ultrasound joint (for effusion, bone destruction). MRI if osteomyelitis suspected.

⨿ Sudden onset of severe monoarthritic:

- ❖ **Implications / Diagnoses:** Septic arthritis (until proven otherwise), Crystal arthropathy (gout or pseudogout), Traumatic hemarthrosis.
- ❖ **Investigations:** Urgent joint aspiration (Gram stain, microscopy for crystals, culture), Serum urate, X-ray (for chondrocalcinosis or erosions), Ultrasound if aspiration is difficult.

⨿ Hot, red, swollen joint (especially single large joint):

- ❖ **Implications / Diagnoses:** Septic arthritis, gout/pseudogout, hemarthrosis, or inflammatory arthritis flare.
- ❖ **Investigations:** Joint aspiration for culture and crystals, FBC, CRP/ESR, blood cultures, X-ray / Ultrasound.

⨿ Rapidly progressive joint destruction or deformity:

- ❖ **Implications / Diagnoses:** Septic arthritis, aggressive rheumatoid arthritis, Charcot (neuropathic) joint. Late-stage psoriatic or erosive osteoarthritis.
- ❖ **Investigations:** X-ray → joint space loss, erosions, MRI for bone marrow and soft tissue, Rheumatoid factor (RF), anti-CCP, Blood cultures if infection suspected.

⨿ Weight loss, night sweats, or constitutional symptoms:

- ❖ **Implications / Diagnoses:** Malignancy-associated arthritis (e.g., paraneoplastic), tuberculous arthritis, chronic infection, Systemic autoimmune disease (e.g., SLE, vasculitis).
- ❖ **Investigations:** FBC, ESR/CRP, autoantibody screen (ANA, dsDNA, ENA), TB screen (QuantiFERON, CXR), Malignancy workup: CXR, PSA, mammogram, CT as indicated.

∏ Polyarthritis with rash, mucosal ulcers, or serositis:
- ❖ **Implications / Diagnoses:** Systemic lupus erythematosus (SLE), vasculitis, reactive arthritis, viral arthritis.
- ❖ **Investigations:** ANA, anti-dsDNA, ENA panel, Viral serology (Parvovirus B19, Hep B/C, HIV), Urinalysis for protein/haematuria (lupus nephritis), CXR / ECHO for serositis.

∏ Back pain, stiffness, or enthesitis with peripheral arthritis:
- ❖ **Implications / Diagnoses:** Spondyloarthropathy (ankylosing spondylitis, psoriatic arthritis, IBD-related).
- ❖ **Investigations:** HLA-B27, X-ray sacroiliac joints (or MRI early), CRP/ESR, screen for psoriasis/IBD/uveitis.

∏ Multiple joint involvement with early morning stiffness > 30 mins:
- ❖ **Implications / Diagnoses:** Inflammatory arthritis (Rheumatoid arthritis, SLE, polymyalgia rheumatica).
- ❖ **Investigations:** RF, anti-CCP, ANA, ESR/CRP, X-ray hands/feet for erosions.

∏ History of recent infection (especially GI/GU) preceding arthritis:
- ❖ **Implications / Diagnoses:** Reactive arthritis (post-Chlamydia, Salmonella, Shigella, Yersinia, Campylobacter).
- ❖ **Investigations:** Urine PCR for Chlamydia, stool culture, HLA-B27, ESR/CRP.

∏ Hemarthrosis or easy bruising:
- ❖ **Implications / Diagnoses:** Coagulopathy, anticoagulant use, trauma, or haemophilia.
- ❖ **Investigations:** PT, aPTT, INR, platelet count, Joint aspiration (if safe), Imaging for internal bleeding.

∏ Pain out of proportion, severe tenderness, or inability to move joint:

- ❖ **Implications / Diagnoses:** Septic arthritis, necrotizing fasciitis, compartment syndrome, or fracture.
- ❖ **Investigations:** Urgent imaging (X-ray/MRI), Blood cultures, CRP/WCC, Surgical referral if infection suspected.

∏ Associated neuropathy, sensory loss, or painless swelling:

- ❖ **Implications / Diagnoses:** Charcot joint (neuropathic arthropathy) due to diabetes, tabes dorsalis, or syphilis.
- ❖ **Investigations:** Neuropathy screen (monofilament, HbA1c, B12), X-ray/MRI → joint destruction, fragmentation.

🗝 Key points:

- **Monoarthritic** → think infection or crystal disease
- **Symmetrical small-joint arthritis** → rheumatoid
- **Asymmetrical large-joint + enthesitis** → spondyloarthritis
- **Morning stiffness duration helps differentiate:**

    <30 min → *mechanical- e.g. Osteoarthritis*
    >30 min → *inflammatory- e.g. RA*

- Check systemic clues: rash, oral ulcers, uveitis, bowel or urinary symptoms.
- Atraumatic joint pain may be associated with degenerative disease, crystal-induced arthropathy, infection, or cancer.
- In cases where a joint presents with redness, warmth, and swelling, joint aspiration is essential to exclude the possibility of infection.
- Osteoarthritis is the most common cause of acute nontraumatic monarthritis in older adults.

- Crystals in synovial fluid confirms crystal-induced arthritis but do not rule out co-existing infection.
- Joint pain that is still unexplained after x-ray and arthrocentesis should be evaluated with MRI to rule out occult fracture, avascular necrosis, synovitis, meniscal/ligament tear.

ABC approach to joint pain and swelling (evaluation + workup):

A — Assessment and immediate threats

Rapid severity check

- Obs/NEWS2, pain severity, ability to weight-bear/use limb, systemic features (fever, rigors), immunosuppression.

Immediate threats / red flags (treat as emergency until excluded)

- **Septic arthritis** (especially **hot, swollen, very painful joint** + fever or systemic upset)
  - Risk ↑: prosthetic joint, RA, diabetes, immunosuppression, IVDU
- **Crystal arthritis with sepsis mimic** (gout/pseudogout can look toxic—still aspirate)
- **Cauda equina / spinal infection** (back pain + fever + neuro deficit) if symptoms are spinal rather than joint
- **Acute neurovascular compromise** (cold limb, absent pulses, severe pain)
- **Fracture/haemarthrosis** (trauma, anticoagulation) esp. unable to weight bear
- **Hot swollen calf + joint symptoms** (DVT or ruptured Baker's cyst—consider VTE if risk)

Immediate actions if septic joint is possible

- **Urgent joint aspiration BEFORE antibiotics** (if feasible and no delay to resus)
- Start **IV antibiotics after cultures/aspirate** (per local guideline)
- Early **orthopaedics/rheumatology** (and micro) input; consider washout
- Analgesia, immobilise, elevate

B — Bedside assessment (focused history and exam)

Focused history

- **Time course:** sudden (hours–days) vs chronic (weeks–months)
- **Pattern: monoarticular vs oligo/polyarticular;** migratory vs additive
- **Inflammatory features:** morning stiffness >30–60 min, night pain, warmth/redness
- **Systemic symptoms:** fever, weight loss, rash, uveitis symptoms, diarrhoea/urethritis
- **Triggers:** trauma, recent infection, new meds (diuretics), alcohol, high purine diet, dehydration
- **PMH:** gout, RA, psoriasis, IBD, CKD, diabetes, immunosuppression, prosthetic joints
- **Infection risks:** skin breaks, recent surgery/injection, IVDU, STI risk
- **Bleeding risk:** anticoagulants, bleeding disorder

Focused exam

- **Vitals** (fever matters)
- **Joint exam:** look-feel-move
    - Effusion, warmth, erythema, tenderness, ROM (active + passive), deformity
- **Compare sides**; check **neurovascular status**
- **Extra-articular signs:**
    - Skin: psoriasis, purpura, erythema nodosum
    - Eyes: red painful eye (uveitis)
    - Mouth ulcers; tophi
- **Adjacent structures:** cellulitis, bursitis, tendonitis
- If calf swelling: assess for **DVT/Baker's** cyst features

C-Core investigations (workup)

Core principle: aspirate any unexplained hot swollen joint

Joint aspiration (synovial fluid)

- **Gram stain & culture**
- **Cell count** (WBC)
- **Crystals** (MSU/CPPD)
- ± glucose/protein per local lab

Baseline bloods (most acute inflammatory presentations)

- **FBC, CRP/ESR**
- **U&E/creatinine**, LFT (baseline + medication planning)
- **Urate** (supportive only—can be normal in acute gout)
- **Blood cultures** if febrile or septic

Imaging

- **X-ray** if trauma, severe pain, suspected fracture, chronic disease, or first presentation of swollen joint
- **Ultrasound** to confirm effusion/guide aspiration (esp. hip/shoulder)
- **MRI** if suspected osteomyelitis, septic focus, or internal derangement and diagnosis unclear

Targeted tests (guided by pattern)

- **Rheumatoid arthritis:** RF, anti-CCP (do not delay aspiration if septic arthritis possible)
- **Spondyloarthritis/reactive arthritis:** consider HLA-B27; screen for **GI/GU infection** (stool tests, chlamydia/gonorrhoea NAAT) if relevant
- **Connective tissue disease/vasculitis:** ANA, complements, urinalysis if systemic features
- **Lyme** only if exposure risk + compatible features

Disposition pointers

- **Suspected septic arthritis** → admit, urgent aspiration + IV antibiotics ± washout
- **Confirmed crystal arthritis** but systemically well → treat; still safety-net if fever/persistent symptoms

Mnemonic for Joint Pain Red Flags — "FRACTURED JOINT"

F – Fever/systemic illness → septic arthritis

R – Rapid swelling/onset → infection or crystals

A – Acute monoarthritis → urgent aspiration

C – Constitutional symptoms → malignancy/TB

T – Trauma or tenderness severe → fracture/hemarthrosis

U – Unexplained weight loss → cancer/infection

R – Rash or ulcers → autoimmune (SLE, vasculitis)

E – Early morning stiffness → inflammatory arthritis

D – Drug use/anticoagulation → hemarthrosis

J – Joint deformity → RA, Charcot

O – On anticoagulants → bleeding into joint

I – Immunosuppression → atypical infection

N – Neuropathy → Charcot joint

T – Tuberculosis / chronic infection sign

Quick Mnemonic – "PAINS"

Pattern (mono vs poly, symmetric vs asymmetric)

Acute vs chronic

Inflammatory signs

Non-articular features (rash, fever, uveitis)

Serology & imaging

Nausea and Vomiting

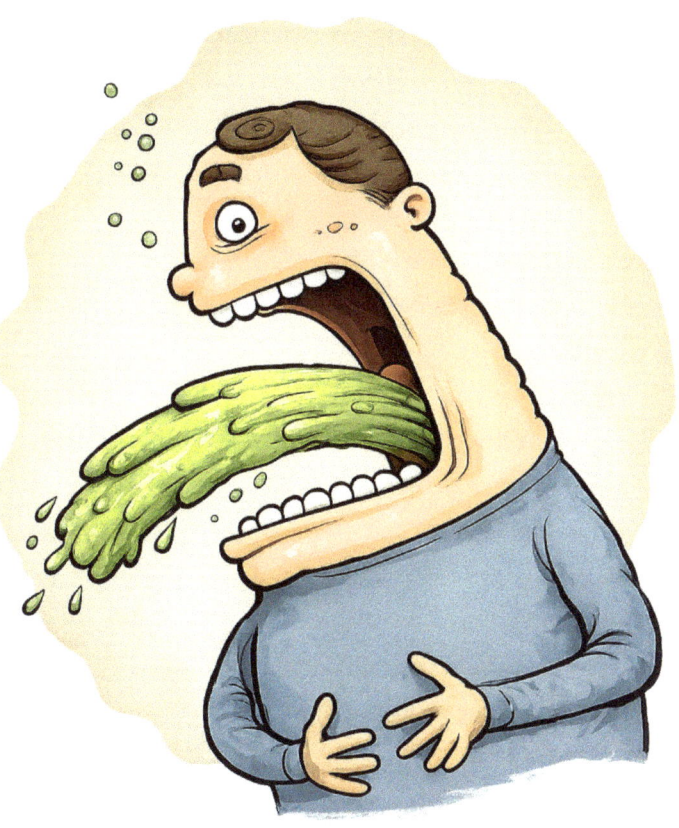

Red Flags: Nausea and vomiting

- ⚠ Haematemesis (vomiting blood)
- ⚠ Projectile vomiting without nausea
- ⚠ Severe abdominal pain, distension, or tenderness
- ⚠ Bilious (green) vomiting
- ⚠ Persistent vomiting with weight loss or early satiety
- ⚠ Neurological symptoms (headache, visual changes, confusion, focal deficits)
- ⚠ Severe dehydration or hypotension
- ⚠ History of recent head injury
- ⚠ Vomiting with severe chest pain or after forceful retching
- ⚠ Pregnancy with severe vomiting (especially before 12 weeks)
- ⚠ Associated jaundice or right upper quadrant pain
- ⚠ Polypharmacy or drug use (especially opioids, digoxin, chemotherapy)
- ⚠ Severe metabolic or endocrine abnormalities
- ⚠ Vomiting that awakens patient at night or is associated with early satiety

∏ Haematemesis (vomiting blood):

- ❖ **Implications / Diagnoses:** Upper GI bleed – peptic ulcer, varices, Mallory-Weiss tear, gastritis, or malignancy. Can be life-threatening if massive or recurrent.

- ❖ **Investigations:** Urgent FBC, U&E, LFTs, coagulation profile., Group & crossmatch., Upper GI endoscopy (diagnostic ± therapeutic), Abdominal ultrasound/CT if varices or malignancy suspected.

∏ Projectile vomiting without nausea:
- ❖ **Implications / Diagnoses:** Pyloric stenosis, Raised intracranial pressure (ICP) - tumour, hydrocephalus, bleed.
- ❖ **Investigations:** Abdominal ultrasound (pyloric stenosis), CT/MRI brain (if raised ICP suspected), Electrolytes – often show hypochloraemia metabolic alkalosis.

∏ Severe abdominal pain, distension, or tenderness:
- ❖ **Implications / Diagnoses:** Bowel obstruction, peritonitis, pancreatitis, or intestinal perforation, Surgical or obstructive cause until proven otherwise.
- ❖ **Investigations:** Abdominal X-ray / CT abdomen-pelvis, Amylase/lipase (pancreatitis). LFTs, U&E, CRP, Urinalysis / pregnancy test in females.

∏ Bilious (green) vomiting:
- ❖ **Implications / Diagnoses:** Intestinal obstruction distal to ampulla of Vater – duodenal, jejunal, or small-bowel obstruction.
- ❖ **Investigations:** Abdominal X-ray (air–fluid levels, distension), CT abdomen, Electrolytes for dehydration/alkalosis.

∏ Persistent vomiting with weight loss or early satiety:
- ❖ **Implications / Diagnoses:** Gastric outlet obstruction, gastric cancer, gastroparesis, Chronic GI or systemic disease (CKD, adrenal insufficiency).
- ❖ **Investigations:** Upper GI endoscopy ± biopsy, Abdominal ultrasound/CT scan, U&E, renal profile, HbA1c, thyroid/adrenal tests.

∏ Neurological symptoms (headache, visual changes, confusion, focal deficits):
- **Implications / Diagnoses:** Raised intracranial pressure, meningitis, encephalitis, intracranial bleed, brain tumour, migraine with aura.
- **Investigations:** CT/MRI brain, Lumbar puncture (if no mass lesion suspected), FBC, CRP, electrolytes.

∏ Severe dehydration or hypotension:
- **Implications / Diagnoses:** Severe gastroenteritis, DKA, Addisonian crisis, hyperemesis gravidarum, intestinal obstruction.
- **Investigations:** U&E, bicarbonate, glucose, ketones, cortisol/ACTH (if Addisonian). Urinalysis, ABG, Pregnancy test (females of reproductive age).

∏ History of recent head injury:
- **Implications / Diagnoses:** Raised ICP, intracranial bleed (subdural, extradural, intracerebral).
- **Investigations:** CT head (non-contrast). FBC, coagulation profile (especially if on anticoagulants).

∏ Vomiting with severe chest pain or after forceful retching:
- **Implications / Diagnoses:** Boerhaave's syndrome (oesophageal rupture) or Mallory-Weiss tear, Surgical emergency (risk of mediastinitis).
- **Investigations:** CXR → mediastinal air, CT chest with contrast / contrast swallow, Urgent surgical review.

∏ Pregnancy with severe vomiting (especially before 12 weeks):
- **Implications / Diagnoses:** Hyperemesis gravidarum – may cause severe dehydration, electrolyte imbalance, and Wernicke's encephalopathy.

- ❖ **Investigations:** Urine ketones, U&E, LFTs, Thiamine levels (before glucose infusion), Ultrasound (confirm pregnancy, exclude molar pregnancy).

∏ Associated jaundice or right upper quadrant pain:
- ❖ **Implications / Diagnoses:** Hepatitis, biliary obstruction, cholecystitis, pancreatitis.
- ❖ **Investigations:** LFTs, amylase/lipase, Abdominal ultrasound / MRCP, Hepatitis screen if indicated.

∏ Polypharmacy or drug use (especially opioids, digoxin, chemotherapy):
- ❖ **Implications / Diagnoses:** Drug-induced nausea (iatrogenic), Digoxin toxicity, opioid effects, chemotherapy-induced nausea.
- ❖ **Investigations:** Drug levels (e.g., digoxin), Renal/liver function tests, Medication review.

∏ Severe metabolic or endocrine abnormalities:
- ❖ **Implications / Diagnoses:** DKA, Addisonian crisis, uraemia, hypercalcaemia, thyrotoxicosis.
- ❖ **Investigations:** U&E, calcium, glucose, ketones, cortisol, TFTs, ABG, Urinalysis.

∏ Vomiting that awakens patient at night or is associated with early satiety:
- ❖ **Implications / Diagnoses:** Raised intracranial pressure, gastric cancer, or ulcer disease.
- ❖ **Investigations:** CT/MRI brain, Upper GI endoscopy.

🗝 Key points:
- **Morning vomiting + headache** → raised ICP (think tumour)

- **Vomiting without nausea** → intracranial cause
- **Bilious vomiting** → distal obstruction
- **Feculent vomiting** → large bowel obstruction
- **Pregnant + vomiting + ketones** → hyperemesis gravidarum
- **Always review drug chart** — many meds cause nausea

ABC approach to nausea and vomiting (evaluation + workup)

A — Assessment and immediate threats

Rapid severity check

- Obs/NEWS2, **hydration**, mental state, urine output, **capillary glucose**, pain score.
- Look for **shock**, sepsis, ongoing profuse vomiting, inability to keep fluids down.

Immediate threats / red flags (urgent same-day / ED)

- **GI obstruction:** severe colicky pain, **distension**, absolute constipation, feculent vomiting
- **GI bleed:** haematemesis/coffee-ground vomit, melaena, syncope
- **Sepsis:** fever/rigors, hypotension, confusion (any source incl. biliary/UTI/abdominal)
- **Acute abdomen/peritonism:** guarding, rebound, rigid abdomen
- **Pancreatitis:** severe epigastric pain radiating to back, persistent vomiting
- **Biliary sepsis/cholangitis:** RUQ pain + fever ± jaundice
- **ACS** (especially older/diabetic): epigastric discomfort, diaphoresis, dyspnoea

- **Raised ICP/CNS infection:** headache, meningism, focal neurology, altered GCS, vomiting on waking
- **DKA/metabolic:** polyuria/polydipsia, Kussmaul breathing, ketones, severe dehydration
- **Toxic ingestion/overdose** (incl. paracetamol) or severe alcohol withdrawal
- **Pregnancy complications / hyperemesis:** dehydration, ketonuria, weight loss

Immediate actions
- IV access, **IV fluids**, antiemetic, analgesia; correct electrolytes
- **NBM** if obstruction/acute abdomen suspected
- Early senior/surgical review if peritonism/obstruction; isolation precautions if infectious outbreak suspected

B — Bedside assessment (focused history and exam)

Focused history
- **Onset & course:** acute vs chronic; frequency; triggers (meals, motion, smells)
- **Character:** bilious? feculent? blood? coffee-ground?
- **Associated symptoms:**
  - Abdominal pain (site/radiation), diarrhoea, constipation, distension
  - Fever, urinary symptoms, headache/photophobia, vertigo
  - Chest pain, breathlessness, palpitations
- **Hydration & intake:** thirst, dizziness, reduced urine, weight loss

- **Pregnancy** possibility; LMP
- **Meds/toxins:** opioids, antibiotics, NSAIDs, GLP-1 agonists, digoxin; alcohol/drugs; recent chemo
- **PMH:** diabetes (DKA), migraines, gallstones, pancreatitis, bowel surgery (adhesions), renal failure, Addison's
- **Exposure:** sick contacts, travel, food poisoning

Focused exam

- **General:** dehydration, cachexia, jaundice, ketotic breath
- Vitals: fever, tachycardia, hypotension
- Abdomen: distension, tenderness, masses, bowel sounds, **peritonism**
- Neuro: GCS, focal deficits, meningism if indicated
- CVS/resp: assess for ACS/HF or aspiration
- Bedside: glucose, urine dip (ketones), bladder scan if retention suspected

C — Core investigations (workup)

Baseline (most moderate–severe, recurrent, or admitted cases)

- **Bloods:** FBC, **U&E/creatinine**, LFTs, CRP, **glucose, calcium** ± magnesium
- **VBG/ABG** + **lactate** if unwell, shocked, suspected DKA/sepsis
- **Urinalysis** (ketones, infection) ± MSU culture if urinary symptoms
- **Pregnancy test** (all women of childbearing potential)
- **ECG** (especially if chest/epigastric pain, electrolyte derangement, or antiemetics affecting QT)

Targeted tests

- **Lipase/amylase** if pancreatitis suspected
- **Troponin** if ACS possible
- **Paracetamol level/toxicology** if overdose possible or unclear history
- **Blood cultures** if febrile/septic

Imaging (based on likely diagnosis)

- **CT abdomen/pelvis** if obstruction, peritonism, severe/unexplained abdominal pain
- **Abdominal X-ray** can support obstruction but CT is usually definitive if concern
- **RUQ ultrasound** if biliary colic/cholecystitis/cholangitis suspected
- **CT head** if red flags for raised ICP/ICH/CNS infection (then LP if indicated and safe)

If you meant **"nausea/vomiting with swelling"** (e.g., facial/leg swelling or abdominal

Mnemonic Summary — "VOMIT"

V – Vestibular / CNS O – Obstruction

M – Metabolic / endocrine

I – Infection / inflammation

T – Toxins / drugs

📕 Mnemonic for Nausea & Vomiting Red Flags — "VOMIT DANGER"

V – Vomiting blood → upper GI bleed

O – Obstruction signs (distension, pain, bilious) → bowel obstruction

M – Meningism / neuro signs → raised ICP or meningitis

I – Intracranial pathology (headache, trauma)

T – Tender abdomen / peritonitis → surgical abdomen

D – Dehydration or hypotension → DKA/Addisonian crisis

A – Associated jaundice → hepatobiliary disease

N – Neurological symptoms → raised ICP / tumour

G – GI outlet obstruction / cancer → persistent vomiting + weight loss

E – Electrolyte or metabolic causes

R – Rupture (Boerhaave's) / pregnancy-related hyperemesis

Palpitations

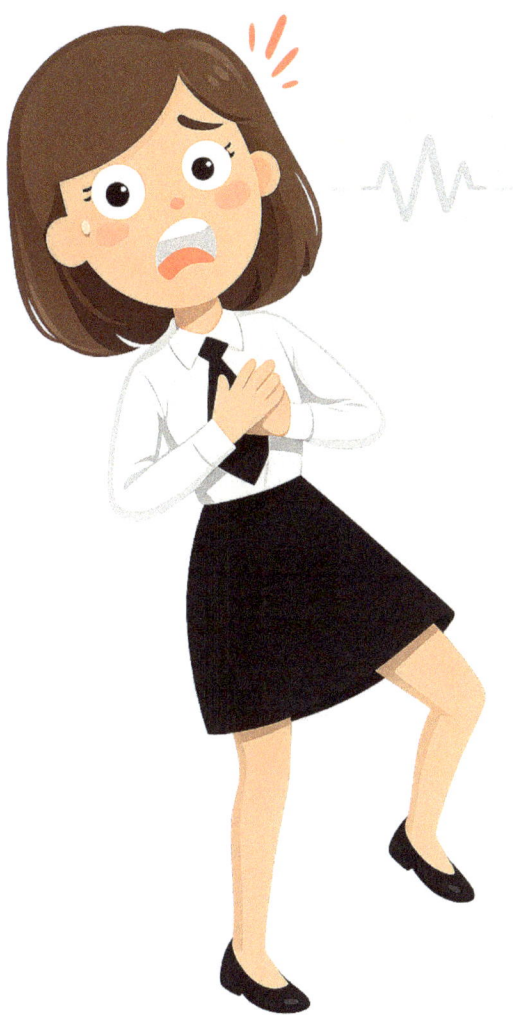

▶ Red Flags: Palpitations

- ⚠ **Syncope or Presyncope**
- ⚠ **Chest Pain or Tightness**
- ⚠ **Dyspnoea, Orthopnoea, or Signs of Heart Failure**
- ⚠ **Exertional Palpitations or Exertional Syncope**
- ⚠ **Family History of Sudden Cardiac Death (<40 yrs)**
- ⚠ **Known Structural or Ischaemic Heart Disease**
- ⚠ **Abnormal ECG Findings**
- ⚠ **Systemic Symptoms (Fever, Weight Loss, Tremor)**

∏ Syncope or Presyncope:

- ❖ **Implications / Diagnoses:** Suggests transient cerebral hypoperfusion, Ventricular tachycardia, high-grade AV block, long QT syndrome. May indicate serious arrhythmia requiring urgent assessment.
- ❖ **Investigations:** 12-lead ECG (QT interval, AV block), 24-hr Holter or event monitor, Echocardiogram, Tilt-table test if reflex syncope suspected.

∏ Chest Pain or Tightness:

- ❖ **Implications / Diagnoses:** Possible myocardial ischaemia precipitated by arrhythmia, AF with rapid ventricular response, SVT, VT secondary to **CAD**.
- ❖ **Investigations:** ECG for ST/T changes, Troponin levels. Echocardiogram. Coronary CT angiography or invasive angiography if needed.

∏ Dyspnoea, Orthopnoea, or Signs of Heart Failure:
- **Implications / Diagnoses:** Suggests impaired cardiac function or tachycardia-induced cardiomyopathy, atrial flutter, or persistent tachyarrhythmia.
- **Investigations:** ECG. BNP or NT-proBNP. Echocardiogram (LV function, valvular disease). Chest X-ray.

∏ Exertional Palpitations or Exertional Syncope:
- **Implications / Diagnoses:** Strong association with malignant arrhythmias. Possible HCM, aortic stenosis, ventricular arrhythmia.
- **Investigations:** ECG., Echocardiogram (LV wall thickness, obstruction), Exercise stress test.

∏ Family History of Sudden Cardiac Death (<40 yrs):
- **Implications / Diagnoses:** Suggests inherited cardiac conditions, Long QT syndrome, Brugada syndrome, HCM, ARVC.
- **Investigations:** ECG (Brugada, long QT, epsilon waves), Echocardiogram, Cardiac MRI, Consider genetic testing.

∏ Known Structural or Ischaemic Heart Disease:
- **Implications / Diagnoses:** Higher risk of ventricular arrhythmias and sudden cardiac death, Post-MI VT, heart failure–related arrhythmia.
- **Investigations:** ECG, Echocardiogram, Cardiac MRI (scar). Holter monitoring.

∏ Abnormal ECG Findings:
- **Implications / Diagnoses:** Indicates underlying arrhythmogenic substrates: prolonged QT, WPW (delta wave), Brugada pattern, VT runs, AV block.

- ❖ **Investigations**, Repeat ECG if needed., Holter/event monitor, Electrophysiology study (if high-risk), Echo or cardiac MRI.

∏ Systemic Symptoms (Fever, Weight Loss, Tremor):
- ❖ **Implications / Diagnoses:** Suggests metabolic, infectious or endocrine causes. Thyrotoxicosis, anaemia, sepsis, hypovolemia.
- ❖ **Investigations:** FBC, CRP/ESR, Thyroid function tests, Electrolytes, renal function, Infection screen if febrile.

🗝 Key points:
- **Most palpitations are benign**, especially ectopic beats, but **always screen for red flags** (syncope, exertional symptoms, chest pain, known heart disease).
- **Character of the rhythm helps:**
    - *Sudden start/stop* → SVT
    - *Irregularly irregular* → AF
    - *Fast, regular, narrow complex* → SVT
    - *Fast, broad complex* → VT (dangerous)
- **Check for reversible triggers:** caffeine, alcohol, nicotine, stress, sleep loss, anaemia, hyperthyroidism, infection, hypoglycaemia, and stimulants (β-agonists, decongestants).
- **Investigate with an ECG first**, then bloods (FBC, U&E, Mg, TSH), and Holter monitoring if episodes are intermittent.
- **Consider echocardiography** if there is any suspicion of structural disease or abnormal baseline ECG.
- **Palpitations with exertion or syncope are red flags** → urgent cardiology review; think VT or structural heart disease.

- **Ectopic are common and often benign;** management is reassurance, lifestyle modification, and sometimes β-blockers.
- **SVT** often responds to vagal manoeuvres; if not, **adenosine** is first line in acute care.
- **AF** requires assessment for rate vs rhythm control and stroke risk (CHA_2DS_2-VASc).
- **Always safety-net:** seek care for syncope, chest pain, breathlessness, sustained palpitations, or new persistent tachycardia.
- Palpitations alone rarely indicate significant arrhythmia, but in patients with structural heart disease or abnormal ECG, they may signal serious underlying disorder requiring investigation.
- An ECG recorded during symptoms is crucial, as a normal ECG recorded during symptoms free interval does not exclude serious disease.
- Many antiarrhythmics may induce arrhythmias themselves.

ABC approach to palpitations (evaluation + workup)

A — Assessment and immediate threats

Rapid severity check

- Obs/NEWS2: HR, BP, SpO_2, RR, temp; conscious level.
- Identify haemodynamic instability (hypotension, chest pain, syncope, shock, pulmonary oedema).

Immediate threats / red flags (urgent same-day / ED)

- **Unstable tachyarrhythmia/bradyarrhythmia:** hypotension, shock, ongoing chest pain, acute HF, altered consciousness
- **Syncope/presyncope** with palpitations (especially exertional)
- **Chest pain** or ECG ischaemia (ACS/demand ischaemia)
- **Wide-complex tachycardia** (treat as VT until proven otherwise)
- **Very fast AF/flutter** with compromise
- **WPW/Pre-excited AF** suspicion (irregular wide-complex very rapid)
- **Family history sudden cardiac death**, known cardiomyopathy, congenital heart disease
- **Electrolyte emergency** (K/Mg/Ca derangement), severe anaemia, thyrotoxicosis
- **Pregnancy** with significant symptoms

Immediate actions

- **12-lead ECG during symptoms** if possible + cardiac monitoring
- IV access; bloods (below)
- If unstable arrhythmia → follow ALS/tachy/brady algorithm (urgent cardioversion/pacing as indicated)

B — Bedside assessment (focused history and exam)

Focused history

- **Onset/offset:** sudden vs gradual; regular vs irregular; duration; frequency

- **Associated symptoms:** chest pain, breathlessness, dizziness, syncope, exercise intolerance
- **Triggers:** exertion, stress, caffeine/energy drinks, alcohol ("holiday heart"), drugs (cocaine), dehydration, fever
- **Past history:** AF, SVT, thyroid disease, structural heart disease, anxiety/panic, OSA
- **Meds:** beta-agonists, decongestants, stimulants, thyroid hormone; QT-prolonging meds
- **Bleeding/anaemia symptoms**, infection symptoms
- **Family history:** sudden death, cardiomyopathy, channelopathies
- Ask patient to **tap out rhythm** (regular vs irregular can help)

Focused exam

- Vitals; assess stability
- **Pulse:** rate, regularity; check for postural drop
- **Cardiac exam:** murmurs (valve disease), signs of HF (JVP, oedema, crackles)
- Thyroid signs (tremor, goitre), anaemia signs, fever/dehydration

C- Core investigations (workup)

Core tests for most

- **12-lead ECG** (repeat if intermittent; compare with old)
- **Bloods:** FBC, **U&E, magnesium, calcium, TSH,** glucose
- **Troponin** if chest pain, ischaemic ECG changes, or prolonged tachyarrhythmia with risk factors

- Consider **CRP** if infection suspected
- **Pregnancy test** where relevant

Capture the rhythm (if ECG normal but symptoms recurrent)
- **Ambulatory monitoring**
  - Daily symptoms → **24–48h Holter**
  - Weekly–monthly → **event monitor**
  - Rare but concerning (syncope) → **implantable loop recorder** consideration
- Patient options: symptom diary; some use validated wearable ECG devices (adjunct, not definitive)

Structural evaluation
- **Echocardiogram if:**
  - Abnormal ECG, murmur, HF signs, known structural disease, recurrent AF/flutter, or high-risk history
- Consider **exercise test** if exertional symptoms/possible ischaemia (per pathway)

When to refer urgently
- Palpitations + **syncope**, exertional onset, family history sudden death, or suspected VT/WPW
- New AF with compromise, very fast rates, or heart failure symptoms

Palpitations: regular, sudden start/stop vs irregular

A) Regular + sudden start/stop (often SVT-type)

Typical descriptors
- "Like a switch," **instant onset and offset**
- **Very fast**, usually **regular**
- May respond to **vagal manoeuvres**
- Often occurs at rest or with caffeine/stress; can recur in episodes

Common causes
- **AVNRT / AVRT (SVT)**
- Atrial tachycardia (less common)
- Occasionally regular flutter (often ~150 bpm if 2:1)

What to look for / do
- Try to get an **ECG during symptoms**
- If stable: consider **vagal manoeuvres**; if terminates and history fits, SVT likely
- Check for **WPW clues** on baseline ECG (short PR, delta wave)
- Arrange **ambulatory monitor** if not captured (event monitor useful if intermittent)

Red flags needing urgent assessment
- Syncope/presyncope, chest pain, severe breathlessness, known structural heart disease
- Broad-complex regular tachycardia (treat as **VT** until proven otherwise)

B) Irregular palpitations (often AF/ectopy)

Typical descriptors
- "Fluttery," "skipping," **uneven** or "all over the place"
- Can be intermittent or sustained
- May be triggered by alcohol ("holiday heart"), infection, thyrotoxicosis

Common causes
- **Atrial fibrillation** (classically irregularly irregular)
- **Ectopics** (PACs/PVCs) — irregular "missed beats"/thumps
- Multifocal atrial tachycardia (esp. COPD), atrial flutter with variable block

What to look for / do
- **12-lead ECG** (and repeat if intermittent)
- Bloods: **TSH**, electrolytes (K/Mg), FBC (anaemia), infection markers if relevant
- If suspected AF: assess **rate**, symptoms, haemodynamic stability; plan anticoagulation risk assessment per pathway
- Use **Holter** if frequent daily; **event monitor** if less frequent

Red flags needing urgent assessment
- Irregular palpitations with **syncope**, hypotension, chest pain, acute HF symptoms
- Very fast AF with compromise, or wide/very rapid irregular rhythm (consider **pre-excited AF/WPW**)

Mnemonic red flags palpitations: **BAD BEAT**

- **B – Breathlessness**
- **A – Acute chest pain**
- **D – Dizziness or syncope**
- **B – Background heart disease**
- **E – ECG changes**
- **A – Arrhythmia family history (SCD <40 yrs)**
- **T – Triggered by exertion**

Syncope

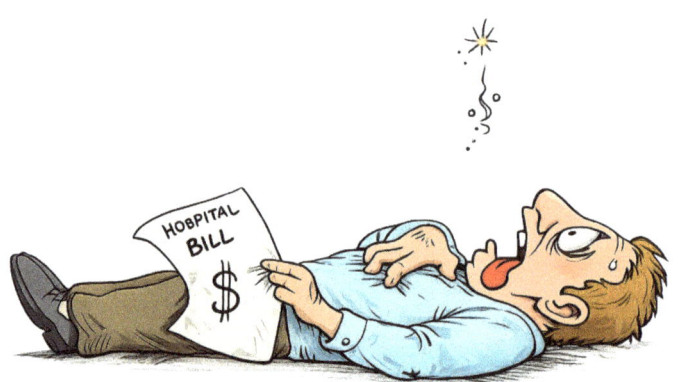

Red Flags: Syncope

- **Syncope During Exertion**
- **Syncope with Chest Pain**
- **Syncope Preceded by Palpitations or Fast Heart Rate**
- **Sudden Syncope Without Warning**
- **Family History of Sudden Cardiac Death Under 40 Years**
- **Syncope While Syncope with Significant Injury, Tongue Biting, or Prolonged Confusion Supine**
- **Abnormal Baseline ECG**
- **Syncope in Known Structural Heart Disease**
- **Multiple recurrences within a short time**

Syncope During Exertion:

- ❖ **Implications/Diagnoses:** Syncope that occurs during exertion suggests a serious underlying cardiac disorder. The most important possibilities include hypertrophic cardiomyopathy, aortic stenosis, arrhythmogenic cardiomyopathy, severe pulmonary hypertension, and exercise-induced ventricular arrhythmias.
- ❖ **Investigations:** The recommended investigations include a 12-lead ECG and an echocardiogram to assess structural heart disease. Exercise ECG testing or cardiology evaluation may be required, and cardiac MRI is useful when the diagnosis remains uncertain or when arrhythmogenic cardiomyopathy is suspected.

∏ Syncope with Chest Pain:

- ❖ **Implications/Diagnoses:** When syncope is associated with chest pain, the concern is that it represents a cardiovascular emergency. The potential diagnoses include acute coronary syndrome, aortic dissection, pulmonary embolism, or ventricular tachyarrhythmias triggered by myocardial ischaemia.
- ❖ **Investigations:** Appropriate investigations include an ECG with serial troponins to detect myocardial ischaemia, along with a chest X-ray. Depending on clinical suspicion, CT aorta may be required when dissection is considered, and CT pulmonary angiography is indicated when pulmonary embolism is a possibility.

∏ Syncope Preceded by Palpitations or Fast Heart Rate:

- ❖ **Implications/Diagnoses:** Syncope that occurs after palpitations or an episode of rapid heart rate raises strong concern for arrhythmias. The possible diagnoses include supraventricular tachycardia, atrial fibrillation, Wolff–Parkinson–White syndrome, ventricular tachycardia, long QT syndrome, and Brugada syndrome. These arrhythmias can cause abrupt drops in cardiac output leading to loss of consciousness.
- ❖ **Investigations:** Investigations should include a detailed ECG with attention to signs such as delta waves, prolonged QT interval, or Brugada patterns. Additional evaluation includes Holter or event monitoring, blood tests for electrolyte abnormalities such as potassium and magnesium, and referral for electrophysiology assessment when necessary.

∏ Sudden Syncope Without Warning:

- **Implications/Diagnoses:** A collapse without any prodromal symptoms is concerning for life-threatening arrhythmias. The main diagnoses include ventricular tachycardia, complete heart block, torsades de pointes, and Stokes–Adams attacks. These events typically occur abruptly and are associated with a high risk of sudden cardiac death.
- **Investigations:** Evaluation includes an ECG, prolonged rhythm monitoring with a 24- to 72-hour Holter, and echocardiography when structural disease is suspected. In some cases, pacemaker assessment or electrophysiology studies may be required.

∏ Family History of Sudden Cardiac Death Under 40 Years:

- Implications/Diagnoses: A family history of young sudden cardiac death suggests inherited arrhythmic or cardiomyopathic conditions. These include long QT syndrome, Brugada syndrome, hypertrophic cardiomyopathy, arrhythmogenic right ventricular cardiomyopathy, and catecholaminergic polymorphic ventricular tachycardia. These conditions often present with fatal arrhythmias in otherwise healthy individuals.
- **Investigations:** Recommended investigations include an ECG to screen for prolonged QT intervals or Brugada patterns, an echocardiogram to assess for cardiomyopathy, and cardiac MRI when ARVC is suspected. Genetic testing may also be considered after cardiology referral.

∏ Syncope While Supine:

- **Implications/Diagnoses:** Syncope occurring while lying down is unusual for benign vasovagal episodes and therefore raises concern for serious arrhythmic events. Potential causes

include ventricular tachycardia, severe bradyarrhythmia, autonomic dysfunction, or rare conditions such as catecholaminergic polymorphic ventricular tachycardia.
- ❖ **Investigations:** The evaluation should include a 12-lead ECG, continuous rhythm monitoring such as Holter recording, and consideration of electrophysiology testing if the episodes are recurrent or unexplained.

∏ Syncope with Significant Injury, Tongue Biting, or Prolonged Confusion:

- ❖ **Implications/Diagnoses:** Syncope associated with major injury, tongue biting, or prolonged post-episode confusion suggests the possibility of a seizure rather than pure syncope, although convulsive syncope may also mimic epilepsy. Distinguishing these conditions is important because the management pathways differ significantly.
- ❖ **Investigations:** Recommended investigations include an ECG, bedside glucose measurement, a neurological examination, and when seizure is strongly suspected, MRI brain and EEG.

∏ Abnormal Baseline ECG:

- ❖ **Implications/Diagnoses:** An abnormal baseline ECG is itself a red flag because it indicates possible underlying electrical or structural heart disease. Relevant abnormalities include long QT intervals, delta waves suggestive of WPW, Brugada type patterns, ventricular ectopy, and various degrees of AV block. These findings increase the likelihood of arrhythmic syncope.
- ❖ **Investigations:** Further evaluation includes repeating the ECG for confirmation, performing an echocardiogram, and arranging Holter monitoring or event recording. Cardiology referral is essential for further risk stratification.

⨅ Syncope in Known Structural Heart Disease:

- ❖ **Implications/Diagnoses:** Patients with established structural heart disease who experience syncope are at high risk for ventricular arrhythmias, reduced cardiac output, or mechanical obstruction. Conditions such as post-MI scar, valve disease, cardiomyopathy, and left ventricular dysfunction are important considerations.
- ❖ **Investigations:** The recommended investigations include an echocardiogram to assess cardiac structure and valve function, a 12-lead ECG, and cardiac MRI when needed for further characterization. An implantable loop recorder may be considered for recurrent, unexplained episodes.

⨅ Multiple recurrences within a short time:

- ❖ **Implications/Diagnoses:** possible Arrhythmias
- ❖ **Investigations:** ECG, Echo, ambulatory ECG, Routine Blood Tests- check for electrolyte abnormalities.

🔑 Key Points:

- Syncope is caused by global CNS dysfunction, typically due to reduced cerebral blood flow.
- Most syncope results from benign causes.
- Rarely, serious causes include cardiac arrhythmia or outflow obstruction.
- Vasovagal syncope is typically associated with an identifiable precipitating factor, prodromal warning signs, and few minutes of residual symptoms following recovery.
- Cardiac arrhythmia-related syncope is sudden with rapid recovery.
- Seizures have a prolonged (e.g hours) recovery period.

- The most common causes are – Vasovagal and idiopathic, many cases never have a firm diagnoses but lead to no apparent harm.
- LOC that is abrupt in onset, is associated with muscular jerking or convulsions, incontinence or tongue biting and is followed by postictal confusion or somnolence suggests a seizure.

CHESS Rule for Syncope:

San Francisco Syncope Rule (SFSR) — "CHESS" (7-day serious outcomes)

Predicts: serious outcomes at **7 days**.

CHESS criteria (any = high risk):

The **CHESS** mnemonic summarises the **five high-risk features** that predict serious outcomes within 7 days after syncope. If **any one** of these is present → the patient is **high-risk**.

C – Congestive Heart Failure

Implications/Diagnoses: History of heart failure increases the likelihood of arrhythmic syncope, low cardiac output states, or decompensation. These patients are more prone to life-threatening events such as ventricular arrhythmias or acute pump failure.

Investigations: ECG to assess for arrhythmias, BNP if fluid overload suspected, and echocardiography (if not recently done) to assess ejection fraction and structural disease.

H – Haematocrit < 30%

Implications/Diagnoses: A low haematocrit points to significant anaemia or acute/chronic blood loss, both of which reduce oxygen delivery and predispose to syncope. It can also indicate underlying GI bleeding or marrow disorder.

Investigations: Full blood count, iron studies or haemolysis markers if needed, and GI work-up (stool testing, endoscopy) if blood loss is suspected.

E – ECG Abnormalities

- **Implications/Diagnoses:** Any abnormal ECG increases suspicion for arrhythmic syncope. This includes conduction blocks (e.g., bundle branch block), ischaemic changes, QT prolongation, arrhythmias, or signs of structural disease.
- **Investigations:** Initial and repeat ECGs, telemetry monitoring, troponin testing, and echocardiography if structural disease is likely.

S – Shortness of Breath

Implications/Diagnoses: Dyspnoea at presentation raises concern for cardiopulmonary causes: heart failure, pulmonary embolism, severe anaemia, or arrhythmias causing poor output.

Investigations: Chest X-ray, BNP, D-dimer/CTPA if PE suspected, and echocardiography to assess cardiac function.

S – Systolic Blood Pressure < 90 mmHg at Triage

Implications/Diagnoses: Hypotension suggests haemodynamic compromise from arrhythmia, shock (cardiogenic, hypovolaemic, or septic), or significant vasovagal reaction with prolonged low output.

Investigations: Serial BP checks, ECG, blood tests (U&E, lactate), and echocardiography if cardiogenic shock or tamponade is suspected.

How to Use CHESS
- **Any CHESS criterion positive → High-risk syncope → Admit / monitor.**
- **No CHESS criteria → Low-risk** but still use clinical judgement (CHESS can miss up to 2–5%).

Canadian Syncope Risk Score (CSRS) — best-validated ED tool (30-day serious outcomes)

Predicts: 30-day serious outcomes after ED assessment/disposition. **Variables (points):**

- Predisposition to vasovagal symptoms (**-1**)
- History of heart disease (**+1**)
- Any SBP reading <**90** or >**180** (**+2**)
- Troponin >99th percentile (**+2**)
- Abnormal QRS axis (**+1**)
- QRS duration >130 ms (**+1**)
- QTc >480 ms (**+2**)
- ED diagnosis: **vasovagal (-2) or cardiac syncope (+2)** **Risk gradient (validation cohort, 30-day serious outcomes):** very low **0.2%**, low **0.7%**, medium **8.0%**, high **19.2%**, very high **51.3%**.

ABC approach to syncope (evaluation + workup):

A — Assessment and immediate threats

First: is this true syncope? (transient loss of consciousness with rapid onset, short duration, complete recovery). If not, consider **seizure, hypoglycaemia, stroke/TIA, intoxication, cataplexy, psychogenic pseudosyncope**.

Immediate red flags = treat as high risk until proven otherwise

- **Airway/breathing compromise**, persistent hypoxia, severe SOB
- **Shock:** SBP <90, cool/clammy, poor perfusion, ongoing syncope/pre-syncope
- **Chest pain / suspected ACS**
- **Palpitations immediately before syncope** (arrhythmic pattern)
- **Abnormal ECG:** bradycardia, high-grade AV block, VT, long QT, WPW pattern, new ischaemia, Brugada pattern
- **Exertional syncope** or syncope **supine**
- **New focal neurology**, severe headache (consider SAH), head injury on anticoagulants
- **GI bleed** symptoms (melaena/haematemesis), severe anaemia
- **Massive PE features** (pleuritic pain, haemoptysis, marked tachycardia, hypoxia, hypotension)

Immediate actions (parallel)

- **ABCDE**, continuous monitoring, **12-lead ECG now**
- **Check capillary glucose**
- **Lying/standing BP** if safe (or after initial stabilisation)
- IV access, bloods, treat causes: fluids if hypovolaemic, manage arrhythmia per ALS, treat anaphylaxis/bleed/PE/ACS as indicated
- If head injury or on anticoagulation: consider urgent imaging based on symptoms/risk

B — Bedside assessment (focused history and exam)

Focused history (high yield)

Event details

- Position (standing/sitting/supine), activity (**exertion?**), setting (hot/crowded), triggers (pain, emotion, coughing, micturition/defecation, shaving)
- Prodrome: nausea, sweating, warmth, visual dimming (vasovagal) vs **sudden with no warning** (arrhythmia)
- Duration of LOC, recovery (rapid recovery suggests syncope; prolonged confusion suggests seizure)
- Witness: pallor, snoring respirations, abnormal movements (brief myoclonic jerks can occur in syncope), tongue biting (lateral), incontinence

Cardiac risk

- Known heart disease/heart failure, congenital disease, family history **sudden cardiac death**
- Palpitations, chest pain, dyspnoea

Volume/medication

- Poor intake, diarrhoea/vomiting, bleeding
- Meds: antihypertensives, diuretics, nitrates, alpha-blockers, QT-prolongers, rate-limiters, alcohol/drugs

Autonomic/orthostatic

- Postural symptoms, neuropathy (diabetes), Parkinsonism, autonomic failure

Focused examination
- **Vitals:** HR, BP, temp, RR, sats; **postural drop** (if safe)
- **Cardiovascular:** murmurs (AS/HCM), signs of HF, irregular pulse, carotid bruits (avoid carotid sinus massage unless specialist setting)
- **Respiratory:** signs of PE/pneumonia
- **Neuro:** focal deficits, postictal state, tongue trauma
- **Hydration/bleeding:** pallor, capillary refill, melaena on PR if indicated

C- Core investigations and workup (baseline for most patients)
- **12-lead ECG** (and rhythm strip if possible)
- **Capillary glucose**
- **Bloods** (tailor): **FBC** (anaemia), **U&E** (electrolytes/renal), **Mg/Ca** if arrhythmia/QT issues, **CRP** if infection suspected
- **Troponin** only if **chest pain/ACS features** or ECG ischaemia (not routinely for all)
- **Pregnancy test** in women of childbearing potential
- **Orthostatic vitals** (lying/standing BP and HR)
- Consider **D-dimer/CTPA** only if PE suspected via clinical probability
- **CXR** if cardiorespiratory symptoms
- **Echocardiography** if murmur/known structural disease/abnormal ECG/heart failure symptoms
- **Ambulatory ECG monitoring** (Holter/event monitor/implantable loop) if intermittent arrhythmia suspected

- **Tilt-table testing** if recurrent unexplained syncope with suspected reflex syncope (usually outpatient)

Mnemonic causes of syncope: **PASS OUT** (Comprehensive syncope causes)

Perfect for recalling the broad categories of causes.

P – Pressure
- Orthostatic hypotension
- Volume depletion
- Vasovagal

A – Arrhythmias
- Bradyarrhythmias
- Tachyarrhythmias

S – Seizures / Neurologic
- Seizure
- Stroke (rare)
- TIA in vertebrobasilar system

S – Sugar
- Hypoglycaemia
- Metabolic causes

O – Output (Cardiac)
- Aortic stenosis
- Hypertrophic cardiomyopathy
- Pulmonary embolism
- Cardiac tamponade

U – Unusual causes
- Medications
- Psychogenic pseudosyncope
- Carotid sinus hypersensitivity

T – Toxins
- Alcohol
- Drugs
- Poisoning

SYNCOPE: mnemonic you can use *for taking a syncope history + spotting red flags*:

S – Situation & trigger
- What were they **doing**? (exertion, standing up, micturition, coughing, pain, emotional stress, hot/crowded room)

Y – sYmptoms before (prodrome)
- Dizziness, nausea, sweating, blurred vision, chest pain, palpitations, aura, focal neuro symptoms?

N – Neurological features
- Tongue bite (lateral), prolonged confusion, incontinence, tonic–clonic movements, focal deficit afterwards → think **seizure / stroke**, not simple syncope.

C – Cardiac clues
- History of IHD, HF, valvular disease, cardiomyopathy, **sudden onset with no warning**, syncope during exertion or when supine, family history of sudden death.

O – Orthostatic & medications
- Postural drop, dehydration, blood loss, antihypertensives, diuretics, vasodilators, rate-limiting drugs.

P – Previous episodes & pattern

- How many episodes, how often, any injuries, worsening pattern, new compared to baseline?

E – ECG & Essentials

- 12-lead ECG (blocks, long/short QT, Brugada, VT, pre-excitation), glucose, Hb, U&E, pregnancy test where relevant.

Orthostatic syncope causes – "DROP"

D – Dehydration

R – Reflex impairment (autonomic failure)

O – Overdose of BP meds

P – Postural drop (≥20/10 mmHg)

The three "P's" are key historical features used to help diagnose uncomplicated vasovagal syncope: **Posture, Provoking factors, and Prodrome**.

- **Posture:** The syncope (fainting) episode typically occurs during prolonged standing or sitting, and the person may have avoided a previous similar episode by lying down.

- **Provoking factors:** There is a clear trigger for the event, such as pain, emotional distress, or a medical procedure (e.g., seeing blood).

- **Prodrome:** The episode is usually preceded by warning symptoms (prodromal symptoms), such as sweating, feeling warm or hot, nausea, dizziness, or "tunnel vision", before the actual loss of consciousness.

Tremor

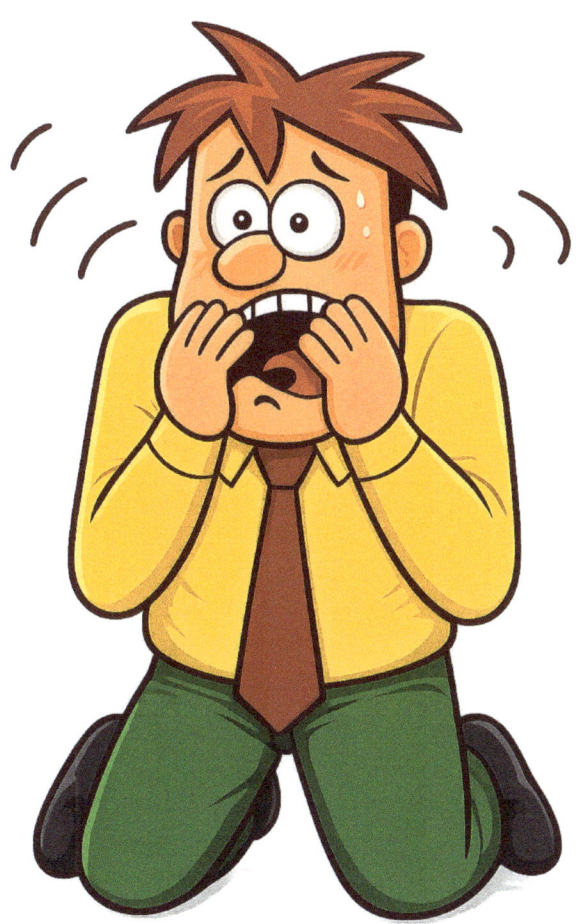

Red Flags: Tremor

- **Acute or Rapidly Progressive Onset**
- **Tremor Associated with Neurological Deficits**
- **Tremor with Cognitive Decline, Behavioral Changes, or Personality Change**
- **Tremor with Rigidity, Bradykinesia, or Resting Tremor**
- **Tremor in a Young Patient (<40 years)**
- **Tremor Triggered or Worsened by New Medications or Substances**
- **Tremor with Abnormal Vital Signs**
- **Tremor Associated with Cerebellar Features (intention tremor, dysmetria, wide-based gait)**
- **Tremor Associated with Liver or Kidney Failure**

Acute or Rapidly Progressive Onset:
- **Implications/Diagnoses:** A tremor that develops suddenly or progresses over days to weeks suggests a secondary cause rather than benign essential tremor. Possible diagnoses include stroke (especially cerebellar), drug-induced tremor, toxic metabolic states, or central nervous system infection.
- **Investigations:** Urgent CT/MRI brain to exclude stroke or mass lesion; drug/toxin screen, metabolic panel (renal, liver, glucose, calcium, magnesium), infection markers.

⌐ Tremor Associated with Neurological Deficits:

- ❖ **Implications/Diagnoses:** Weakness, ataxia, dysarthria, diplopia, abnormal reflexes, or sensory loss point toward Parkinson's disease, multiple sclerosis, cerebellar lesions, Wilson disease, or brainstem pathology.
- ❖ **Investigations:** MRI brain and spine, neurology examination, copper/ceruloplasmin for Wilson disease in young patients, TFTs, B12, autoimmune screen if MS suspected.

⌐ Tremor with Cognitive Decline, Behavioral Changes, or Personality Change:

- ❖ **Implications/Diagnoses:** Suggests neurodegenerative disease such as Parkinson's disease dementia, Lewy body dementia, or frontotemporal disorders.
- ❖ **Investigations:** MoCA or cognitive testing, MRI brain, DAT-scan if uncertainty between Parkinsonian vs non-Parkinsonian tremor.

⌐ Tremor with Rigidity, Bradykinesia, or Resting Tremor:

- ❖ **Implications/Diagnoses:** These cardinal Parkinsonian signs indicate Parkinson's disease, Parkinson-plus syndromes (MSA, PSP, CBD), or drug-induced parkinsonism from antipsychotics or metoclopramide.
- ❖ **Investigations:** Neurology assessment, DAT-scan to confirm dopaminergic deficit, review of medication history.

⌐ Tremor with Autonomic Instability or Systemic Illness:

- ❖ **Implications/Diagnoses:** Tremor accompanied by fever, confusion, hypertension, tachycardia, diaphoresis, or agitation may indicate thyrotoxicosis, sepsis, serotonin syndrome, neuroleptic malignant syndrome, pheochromocytoma, or alcohol withdrawal.

- **Investigations:** TFTs, infection screen, CK, drug screen, urine/plasma metanephrines, alcohol level, electrolytes, EKG.

∏ Tremor in a Young Patient (<40 years):
- **Implications/Diagnoses:** Unusual age of onset raises suspicion for Wilson disease, dystonic tremor, genetic degenerative disorders, or drug-induced tremor.
- **Investigations:** Ceruloplasmin, 24-hour urinary copper, liver function tests, Kayser–Fleischer ring exam, MRI brain, genetic testing if dystonia suspected.

∏ Tremor Triggered or Worsened by New Medications or Substances:
- **Implications/Diagnoses:** Common culprits include β-agonists, SSRIs/SNRIs, lithium, valproate, stimulants, antipsychotics, steroids, caffeine, and recreational drugs.
- **Investigations:** Full medication review, drug screen, renal/liver tests to exclude accumulation toxicity, lithium level if relevant.

∏ Tremor with Abnormal Vital Signs:
- **Implications/Diagnoses:** Hypertension, tachycardia, pyrexia, or tachypnoea may point to endocrine, toxic, or infective causes such as thyrotoxicosis, DKA, or withdrawal syndromes.
- **Investigations:** TFTs, glucose/ketones, arterial blood gas, electrolytes, infection markers.

∏ Tremor Associated with Cerebellar Features (intention tremor, dysmetria, wide-based gait):
- **Implications/Diagnoses:** Suggests cerebellar stroke, multiple sclerosis, alcohol-related cerebellar disease, brain tumours, or drug toxicity (e.g., anticonvulsant toxicity).

- ❖ **Investigations:** MRI brain, especially posterior fossa; alcohol level, antiepileptic drug levels, autoimmune screen if MS suspected.

∏ Tremor Associated with Liver or Kidney Failure:
- ❖ **Implications/Diagnoses:** Flapping tremor (asterixis) indicates hepatic encephalopathy, uraemic encephalopathy, hypercapnia, or toxin accumulation.
- ❖ **Investigations:** LFTs, ammonia, renal panel, ABG, lactate, toxin screen.

🔑 Key Points:
- MRI or CT brain should be done if-Tremor onset is acute, progression is rapid, neurologic signs suggests stroke, a demyelinating disorder or a structural lesion.
- The most common causes of tremor include physiologic tremor, essential tremor and Parkinson's disease.
- Abrupt onset of tremor or tremor in patients who are < 50 and do not have a family history of benign tremor requires prompt, in-depth evaluation.
- Drugs can cause or aggravate different types of tremor.

ABC approach to tremor (evaluation + workup):

A — Assessment and immediate threats

Goal: spot life-threatening/toxic/metabolic causes and "can't miss" neuro emergencies.

1) Rapid triage (first 1–2 minutes)
- **Vitals** (BP, HR, temp, O2 sats) + **capillary glucose**
- **Mental state** (agitation, confusion, delirium)

- **Red flags** → urgent senior/ED/neurology:
  - **Acute onset** (minutes–hours) especially with **focal neurology**, severe headache, ataxia → **stroke/ICH**
  - **Fever, rigidity, autonomic instability** → **serotonin syndrome / NMS / sepsis**
  - **Alcohol withdrawal** (tremor + sweating, tachycardia, hypertension, hallucinations, seizures)
  - **Thyroid storm** (marked tachycardia, hyperthermia, agitation)
  - **Severe hypoglycaemia** or **severe electrolyte disturbance**
  - **Toxic ingestion** (lithium, valproate, stimulants, salicylates, theophylline, etc.)

2) Immediate actions if suspected

- **Hypoglycaemia** → treat immediately (don't wait for labs)
- **Withdrawal** → start protocol (benzodiazepines per local guidance + thiamine if alcohol misuse)
- **Suspected serotonin syndrome/NMS** → stop culprit drugs, supportive care, urgent escalation
- **Sepsis/meningitis/encephalitis** features → sepsis bundle, cultures, antibiotics per pathway
- **Severe hypertension + neuro signs** → emergency pathway

B — Bedside assessment (focused history & exam)

Focused history (high-yield questions)

Characterise the tremor

- **When does it occur?**
    - **Rest tremor** (at rest, improves with action) → Parkinsonism
    - **Postural tremor** (arms outstretched) → essential tremor, drugs, hyperthyroid
    - **Action/kinetic/intention tremor** (worse with movement/targeting) → cerebellar
- **Onset & progression**
    - Sudden onset → drugs/tox/metabolic, stroke, functional tremor
    - Gradual progression → essential tremor, Parkinson's, neuropathic causes
- **Distribution:** hands, head/voice (essential tremor), legs/jaw, unilateral vs bilateral
- **Triggers:** caffeine, stress, fatigue, exertion; **improves with alcohol** (classic essential tremor)

Associated symptoms

- **Parkinsonism:** bradykinesia, rigidity, shuffling gait, micrographia, anosmia, constipation, REM sleep behaviour disorder
- **Cerebellar:** ataxia, dysarthria, nystagmus, wide-based gait
- **Hyperthyroid:** weight loss, heat intolerance, palpitations
- **Withdrawal/toxicity:** sweating, agitation, hallucinations, seizures

- **Neuropathy:** numbness, proprioceptive loss (sensory ataxia)

Medication/substance review (biggest yield)

- **Beta-agonists** (salbutamol), **SSRIs/SNRIs**, antipsychotics, lithium, valproate, stimulants, caffeine, steroids, thyroxine excess
- **Alcohol:** last drink, daily units; benzodiazepine withdrawal; recreational drugs

Background

- Family history (essential tremor)
- Liver/renal disease (asterixis/uraemia), thyroid disease
- Occupational impact (writing, eating, work safety)

Focused examination (bedside)

Observe first

- Tremor **at rest**, **posture** (arms out), **action** (finger-nose), **spiral drawing/writing**, pouring water
- **Frequency** (fine vs coarse), **amplitude**, **distractibility/entrainment** (functional tremor clues)

Neurological exam

- **Parkinsonism:** bradykinesia (finger taps), rigidity (cogwheel), reduced arm swing, masked facies
- **Cerebellar:** dysmetria, intention tremor, rebound, heel-shin, gait ataxia, nystagmus
- **Upper motor neuron signs** or focal deficits → urgent neuroimaging consideration

- **Sensory:** vibration/proprioception, Romberg (sensory ataxia)
- **Asterixis:** "flapping" with wrists extended (hepatic/uraemic/CO_2 retention)

General exam
- **Thyrotoxicosis signs:** tremor, warm hands, goitre, lid lag
- **Autonomic signs:** sweating, tachycardia (withdrawal/tox)
- **Liver disease/renal failure** stigmata

C- Core investigations (workup)

Baseline tests (most patients)
- **Glucose**
- **FBC**
- **U&Es + Ca/Mg**
- **LFTs**
- **TSH + free T4**
- **B12/folate** (if neuropathy/ataxia features)
- **CRP** if infection/systemic illness suspected
- **Drug levels** where relevant: **lithium, valproate, theophylline**; consider **toxicology screen** if unclear

Targeted tests
- **ECG** (tachyarrhythmia, thyrotoxicosis, stimulant effect)
- **ABG/VBG** if hypercapnia suspected (asterixis/CO_2 retention)
- **Ceruloplasmin** + urinary **copper if young** with tremor/dystonia/psychiatric features (Wilson's)

Imaging / specialist tests (based on findings)

- **CT/MRI brain** if **acute onset**, focal deficits, cerebellar signs, severe headache, malignancy/immunosuppression
- **DaTscan** only when diagnosis (ET vs Parkinsonism) remains uncertain after specialist assessment
- Consider **neurology referral** if atypical, rapidly progressive, or treatment-refractory

Mnemonic for Causes of Tremor — "TREMORS"

T – Thyroid & Toxicity

(Thyrotoxicosis, caffeine, alcohol withdrawal, drug toxicity)

R – Rubral & Cerebellar Lesions

(Stroke, MS, tumours, ataxia)

E – Essential Tremor

(Primary familial tremor)

M – Medications

(SSRIs, lithium, valproate, β-agonists, antipsychotics, steroids)

O – Overload / Metabolic

(Hypoglycaemia, hepatic failure with asterixis, renal failure, electrolyte derangements)

R – Resting Tremor / Parkinsonism

(Parkinson's disease, Parkinson-plus syndromes)

S – Stress & Sympathetic Activation

(Anxiety, panic, phaeochromocytoma)

📋 Mnemonic for Tremor Red Flags — "SHAKES"

S – Sudden onset
(stroke, toxins, drugs)

H – Hard neurological signs
(weakness, ataxia, dysarthria → cerebellar/MS/tumour)

A – Age <40 with new tremor
(Wilson disease, genetic disorders)

K – Key systemic signs
(Fever, tachycardia, hypertension → thyrotoxicosis, serotonin syndrome)

E – Escalating progression
(rapid worsening suggests structural or toxic cause)

S – Suspicious medication history
(SSRIs, lithium, valproate, antipsychotics, β-agonists)

Vision loss

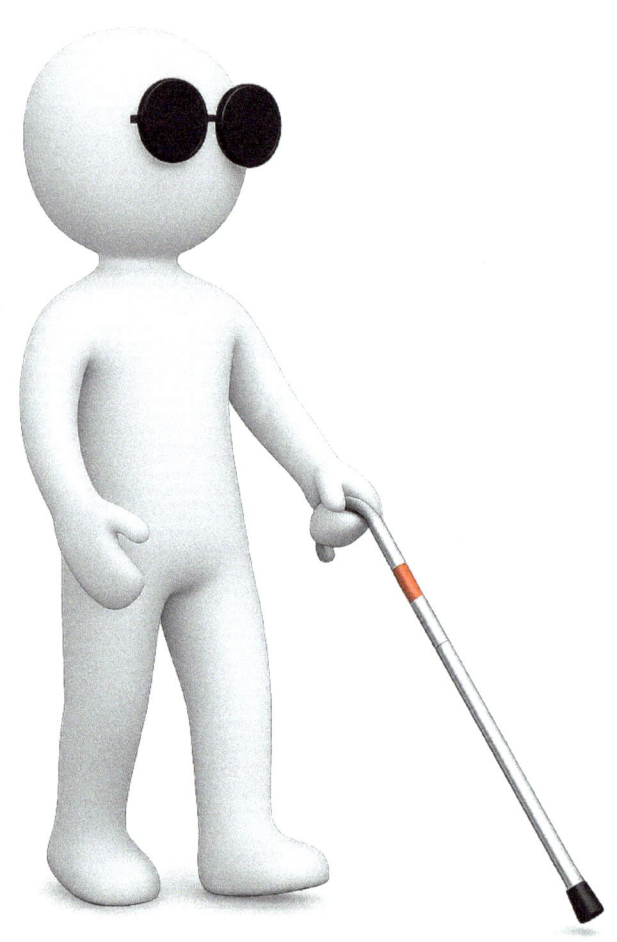

▶ Red Flags: Vision loss

- ⚠ Sudden or rapidly progressive visual loss
- ⚠ Tremor Associated with Neurological Deficits
- ⚠ Painful visual loss or red photophobic eye
- ⚠ Flashes, floaters, "curtain" or shadow
- ⚠ Headache, jaw/temple pain or systemic symptoms in age >50
- ⚠ Visual loss with focal neurological symptoms
- ⚠ Marked asymmetry, RAPD or color desaturation
- ⚠ Bilateral visual loss or visual loss in an only-seeing eye
- ⚠ Transient visual obscurations with features of raised ICP

∏ Sudden or rapidly progressive visual loss:

- ❖ **Implications / diagnoses:** Visual loss over **seconds to hours** or rapidly worsening over hours–days suggests **vascular or acute inflammatory** causes such as **central retinal artery occlusion (CRAO), central retinal vein occlusion (CRVO), ischaemic optic neuropathy, optic neuritis, acute macular pathology, stroke involving the visual pathways**.
- ❖ **Investigations / actions:** Immediate **visual acuity, pupillary responses (RAPD), visual fields**, and **fundoscopy**. Arrange **urgent ophthalmology** review. If stroke suspected, activate **stroke pathway** with **urgent CT/MRI brain ± vascular imaging**.

∏ Painful visual loss or red photophobic eye:

- ❖ **Implications / diagnoses:** Visual loss with **eye pain,** especially **pain on eye movement** or associated **redness/ photophobia,** suggests **optic neuritis, acute angle-closure glaucoma, keratitis/corneal ulcer, anterior uveitis/iritis, scleritis, endophthalmitis,** or **traumatic injury.** These can threaten both sight and sometimes life (e.g. severe infection)

- ❖ **Investigations / actions:** Check **visual acuity, pupils, IOP** (if trained and equipment available), and inspect for **corneal defects** (fluorescein), hypopyon, ciliary injection. Urgent **ophthalmology**; for suspected glaucoma, **immediate ED/ eye casualty**. Take **systemic obs** and consider **blood cultures / inflammatory markers** if infection or systemic autoimmune disease suspected.

∏ Flashes, floaters, "curtain" or shadow:

- ❖ **Implications / diagnoses:** Sudden onset **flashes of light**, new or numerous **floaters**, or a **curtain/veil/shadow** over part of the vision is highly suggestive of **retinal tear or retinal detachment**, or **vitreous haemorrhage/posterior vitreous detachment**, which can very quickly cause permanent visual loss.

- ❖ **Investigations / actions:** Urgent same-day **ophthalmology** for **dilated fundus examination**. If the view to the retina is poor, they may perform **B-scan ocular ultrasound**. Advise the patient to **avoid driving** and keep nil by mouth if surgery likely.

∏ **Headache, jaw/temple pain or systemic symptoms in age >50:**
- ❖ **Implications / diagnoses:** Visual loss with **new headache, scalp tenderness, jaw claudication**, proximal **myalgia/stiffness**, malaise, or low-grade fever in someone **>50 years** is classic for **giant cell arteritis (GCA)** causing **arteritic anterior ischaemic optic neuropathy**. This is an ophthalmic and stroke emergency; the other eye is at high risk.
- ❖ **Investigations / actions**: Treat as **clinical emergency:** start **high-dose steroids immediately** (usually IV then high-dose oral) **without waiting** for tests if suspicion is high. Order urgent **ESR, CRP, FBC, LFTs** and arrange **temporal artery ultrasound** ± **biopsy. Urgent ophthalmology** and usually **rheumatology** input.

∏ **Visual loss with focal neurological symptoms:**
- ❖ **Implications / diagnoses:** Visual loss plus **weakness, numbness, dysarthria, facial droop, ataxia, altered consciousness, seizures** or **homonymous visual field defects** strongly suggests **stroke, TIA, intracranial haemorrhage, brain tumour**, or sometimes **demyelinating disease (e.g. MS)**.
- ❖ **Investigations / actions:** Activate **stroke protocol:** urgent **CT/MRI brain, vascular imaging** (CT angiography/MR angiography/carotid Doppler), ECG and routine stroke bloods. For demyelination, **MRI brain and orbits with contrast**. Always document **visual fields, acuity** and **fundoscopy**.

∏ Marked asymmetry, RAPD or color desaturation:

* **Implications / diagnoses:** A **relative afferent pupillary defect (RAPD)**, or **disproportionate colour vision loss** (e.g. red looks washed-out) compared with acuity, suggests **optic nerve pathology** such as **optic neuritis, ischaemic optic neuropathy, compressive lesions (tumour, aneurysm), or advanced glaucoma**.
* **Investigations / actions:** Perform **pupillary examination, Ishihara colour plates**, and **visual fields**. Urgent **ophthalmology or neuro-ophthalmology** referral. They may request **MRI brain and orbits with contrast**, and **OCT** and **visual evoked potentials** as needed.

∏ Bilateral visual loss or visual loss in an only seeing eye:

* **Implications / diagnoses:** Any significant change in vision in someone with **only one functioning eye**, or **sudden bilateral visual loss**, is automatically a red flag, as the patient may rapidly become functionally blind. Causes include **bilateral optic neuropathies, bilateral occipital lobe stroke, toxic/nutritional optic neuropathy, severe papilloedema/raised ICP, severe bilateral eye disease.**
* **Investigations / actions:** Urgent **ophthalmology** and often **neurology**. Full **neuro-ophthalmic exam, fundoscopy, neuroimaging (CT/MRI)**, and systemic investigations (e.g. for toxins, nutritional deficiency, inflammatory/infective causes) as indicated.

∏ Transient visual obscurations with features of raised ICP:

* **Implications / diagnoses:** Brief episodes of visual blurring or "grey-outs", especially on **bending, coughing or standing**, associated with **morning headache, nausea/vomiting, pulsatile tinnitus**, can represent **raised intracranial pressure** from a

space-occupying lesion, idiopathic intracranial hypertension, venous sinus thrombosis, or other intracranial pathology.

- ❖ **Investigations / actions:** Check **visual acuity, fields**, and look for **papilloedema** on fundoscopy. Arrange **urgent neuroimaging (MRI/CT brain ± MR/CT venography)** before considering lumbar puncture. Early **neurology and ophthalmology** involvement is important.

🗝️ **Key Points:**

- Treat acute visual loss as a **stroke equivalent**.
- If it's sudden onset over seconds–minutes, **think** vascular until proven otherwise **(CRAO, occipital stroke, ischaemic optic neuropathy). Do** a stroke-style assessment: **onset time, neurological symptoms, AF, vascular risk, BP, GCS.**
- **Always ask:** painful or painless? This single question narrows the field massively.
    - **Painful visual loss** → optic neuritis, angle-closure glaucoma, uveitis, keratitis, scleritis, trauma.
    - **Painless visual loss** → CRAO/CRVO, macular disease, GCA, stroke, vitreous haemorrhage, retinal detachment.
- **Check visual acuity properly** – in each eye. Use a Snellen or phone chart if needed. Test **each eye separately** (the good eye can mask profound unilateral loss). Record with pinhole if possible and **document** (e.g. 6/6, 6/12).
- Never skip the **pupils + RAPD**
    - Compare direct and consensual responses.
    - A **relative afferent pupillary defect (RAPD)** = optic nerve / severe retinal disease on that side (optic neuritis, CRAO, severe detachment).

- RAPD is a **big red flag** for urgent specialist review.
- Look for **red eye** + **photophobia** + corneal changes

If it's **red AND painful AND vision ↓**, think **sight-threatening anterior segment pathology:**
- Acute angle-closure glaucoma (rock-hard eye, mid-dilated fixed pupil, haloes).
- Keratitis / corneal ulcer (fluorescein staining, contact lens user).
- Iritis/uveitis (ciliary flush, small pupil). These need **same-day ophthalmology**.

- **Don't miss GCA in anyone >50 with visual symptoms-Ask** headache, scalp tenderness, jaw claudication, PMR symptoms, weight loss. **If suspicious:**
  - **Start high-dose steroids immediately**, then do ESR/CRP, temporal artery US/biopsy.
  - Don't wait for bloods before treating – vision in the other eye is at risk.
- **"Flashes, floaters, curtain" = assume retinal detachment**
Classic story: **new floaters**, **flashing lights**, or a **curtain/veil** coming over vision. Even if some vision remains, this is an **urgent eye casualty** problem – aim same day.
- **Always do a quick neuro screen and visual fields**
  - Check for **homonymous field defects**, neglect, other focal neurology.
  - Any visual loss with **weakness, speech disturbance, ataxia, confusion** → **stroke call** and imaging.
- **Check both BP and glucose in everyone**

Super basic but easy to forget.
- Severe hypertension can come with retinal changes / papilloedema.

- Hypo/hyperglycaemia can present with visual symptoms and confusion.

- **Fundoscopy: even a limited look is better than none**

  You won't always get a perfect view, but try:
  - Swollen disc / blurred margins → papilloedema/optic neuritis.
  - Pallid disc → ischaemic optic neuropathy (think GCA).
  - Cherry red spot → CRAO.

  If you can't see, **say that you tried** and escalate; don't just omit it.

- **Visual loss in an only-seeing eye = automatic emergency**

  Even "mild" symptoms in the **good eye** of someone with poor contralateral vision should be treated as **vision-threatening** until cleared by ophthalmology.

- **Early phone call beats perfect documentation**

- If your gut says "this is bad" (sudden drop, RAPD, red painful eye, GCA features, new neurological signs):

  Call ophthalmology / stroke team early, then complete the clerking.

- **The most common causes of acute loss of vision are:** vascular occlusions of the retina (CRAO, CRVO), Ischemic optic neuropathy (often in patients with temporal arteritis), Vitreous haemorrhage (caused by diabetic retinopathy or trauma), trauma.

- In patients with **binocular, symmetric visual field defects**, consider a lesion of the visual pathways posterior to the optic chiasm.

ABC approach to visual loss (evaluation + workup):

A — Assessment and immediate threats

First, treat as time-critical until proven otherwise (eye + brain).

1) Immediate "can't miss" diagnoses (minutes–hours)

- **Central retinal artery occlusion (CRAO):** sudden, painless, profound monocular loss ("curtain").
- **Acute angle-closure glaucoma:** painful red eye, halos, headache, nausea/vomiting.
- **Giant cell arteritis (GCA):** age >50, headache, scalp tenderness, jaw claudication, systemic symptoms.
- **Retinal detachment:** flashes/floaters + "shadow/curtain".
- **Endophthalmitis / severe keratitis** (esp. contact lens): painful, photophobia, reduced vision.
- **Stroke/TIA/occipital infarct:** homonymous field loss, neuro deficits.
- **Pituitary apoplexy:** sudden headache + visual field defect/ophthalmoplegia.

2) Rapid safety checks (do immediately)

- **Vitals + glucose**
- **Vision "baseline" now:** visual acuity (each eye), pupils (RAPD), visual fields by confrontation.
- **Pain/redness?** → think glaucoma/keratitis/uveitis/endophthalmitis.
- **Monocular vs binocular** (binocular often neuro/occipital; monocular often ocular/retinal/optic nerve).

- **Trauma/chemical exposure?**
  - **Chemical injury: irrigate immediately** (don't wait) until neutral pH, remove contact lenses/particulate matter.

3) Urgent actions while arranging same-day specialty help

- **Suspected GCA:** start **high-dose steroids immediately** (do not wait for ESR/CRP) + urgent ophthalmology/rheum.
- **Suspected acute angle-closure glaucoma:** urgent ophthalmology + start pressure-lowering therapy per local protocol.
- **Suspected CRAO / TIA equivalent:** urgent stroke/eye pathway + vascular risk management.
- **Painful contact lens wearer:** treat as **microbial keratitis until proven otherwise** → urgent ophthalmology, avoid patching.

B — Bedside assessment (focused history & exam)

Focused history (high-yield questions)

- **Onset & tempo:** sudden vs progressive; seconds/minutes vs hours/days.
- **Pain:** none (CRAO/retinal detachment) vs severe (glaucoma/keratitis/uveitis).
- **Laterality:** one eye vs both; **transient vs persistent** (amaurosis fugax).
- **Visual phenomena:**
  - **Flashes/floaters** (retinal tear/detachment, vitreous haemorrhage)
  - **Halos** (glaucoma)

- ○ **Distortion/central blur** (macula)
- ○ **Field defect** (neuro/retinal)
- **Associated symptoms:** headache, jaw claudication, scalp tenderness (GCA); neuro deficits (stroke); fever (infection).
- **Risk factors:** age >50, AF, carotid disease, diabetes, HTN, migraine, autoimmune disease.
- **Eye-specific:** contact lenses, recent surgery/injection, trauma, chemical splash, steroid use.
- **Drug/toxin:** anticholinergics (glaucoma trigger), PDE5 inhibitors (rare NAION association), methanol (toxic optic neuropathy).

Focused examination (bedside)

- **Visual acuity** (with pinhole if available), **colour vision** (red desaturation), **pupils** (RAPD).
- **Visual fields** by confrontation.
- **External eye:** lid swelling, discharge, corneal haze/ulcer, conjunctival injection pattern.
- **Ocular motility + ptosis** (CN palsies, orbital apex/cavernous sinus).
- **Fundoscopy** (if possible):
  - ○ pale retina/cherry red spot (CRAO)
  - ○ swollen disc (papilloedema/optic neuritis/NAION)
  - ○ retinal haemorrhages/"blood and thunder" (CRVO)
  - ○ detachment folds/tear (retinal detachment)
- **If you have access: IOP** (tonometry) and **slit lamp/fluorescein** (abrasion/keratitis).

C- Core investigations (workup)
Minimum in ED/acute medical setting
- **Capillary glucose**
- **ECG** (AF/arrhythmia if vascular cause suspected)
- **Bloods** (tailor to scenario):
  - **ESR + CRP + FBC** (especially if GCA possible)
  - **U&Es, glucose/HbA1c, lipids** (vascular risk)
  - **Coag profile** if haemorrhage/anticoagulation issues
- **Imaging/referrals (based on pattern)**
  - **Suspected stroke/TIA/occipital cause:** urgent neuroimaging per pathway (CT/CTA or MRI)
  - **CRAO/amaurosis fugax: carotid imaging** + cardioembolic workup per local TIA service
  - **Pituitary apoplexy:** urgent endocrine + MRI pituitary (or CT if unstable)
- **Eye-directed tests (often via ophthalmology)**
  - **Ocular ultrasound (B-scan)** if vitreous haemorrhage obscures fundus / retinal detachment suspected
  - **OCT** for macula/optic nerve pathology
  - **Temporal artery ultrasound/biopsy** for GCA confirmation (after steroids started)

📖 Mnemonic for red flags of acute visual loss: **SUDDEN EYE**

S – Sudden onset

Vision loss over seconds to hours or rapidly worsening = assume vascular / acute pathology.

U – Unilateral severe loss / only eye

Markedly worse in one eye, or affecting the only seeing eye → emergency.

D – Discomfort / pain in or around the eye

Especially pain on eye movement → think optic neuritis, acute glaucoma, uveitis, keratitis, scleritis.

D – Dim, red, photophobic eye

Red + painful + ↓ vision = sight-threatening anterior segment disease (glaucoma, keratitis, uveitis, endophthalmitis).

E – Elderly with headache / jaw / scalp pain

Age >50 with visual symptoms + headache, scalp tenderness, jaw claudication, PMR symptoms → giant cell arteritis.

N – Neurological symptoms

Any weakness, numbness, dysarthria, ataxia, confusion, homonymous field loss → think stroke / intracranial lesion.

E – Entoptic phenomena: flashes, floaters, curtain

New flashes, floaters, or a curtain/veil over vision → suspect retinal tear/detachment or VH.

Y – You find RAPD or colour desaturation

RAPD or washed-out red colours → optic nerve / severe retinal disease.

E – Elevated ICP features

Transient visual obscurations, papilloedema, morning headache, vomiting, pulsatile tinnitus → raised ICP.

📋 Mnemonic for acute visual loss: **VISION**

V – Vascular

Sudden, usually **painless** loss

- **C**entral **R**etinal **A**rtery **O**cclusion (CRAO)
- **C**entral **R**etinal **V**ein **O**cclusion (CRVO)
- **Ischaemic optic neuropathy** (incl. GCA)
- **Occipital stroke / TIA** affecting visual pathways

I – Inflammatory / Infective

Often **painful**, red or photophobic eye

- **Optic neuritis**
- **Uveitis / iritis**
- **Keratitis / corneal ulcer** (esp. contact lens wearers)
- **Scleritis**
- **Endophthalmitis** (post-op / post-trauma)

S – Structural retinal / media problems

Physical damage to retina or visual axis

- **Retinal detachment / retinal tear**
- **Vitreous haemorrhage**
- **Macular haemorrhage / macular hole**
- **Trauma** (globe rupture, contusion, lens dislocation)

I – Increased pressure

Pressure-related visual loss

- **Acute angle-closure glaucoma**
- **Raised intracranial pressure** with papilloedema

- **Orbital compartment syndrome** (retrobulbar haematoma)

O – Obstruction of the ocular media

Something blocking light getting to the retina

- **Corneal oedema / opacification** (e.g. severe keratitis, acute glaucoma)
- Dense **cataract** with sudden decompensation (usually more subacute)
- **Hyphaema / hypopyon**
- **Vitreous opacities** (dense VH, endophthalmitis)

N – Neurological

Post-retinal / brain causes

- **Optic nerve compression** (tumour, aneurysm, inflammation)
- **Occipital lobe stroke / tumour**
- **Migraine aura** (usually transient, often positive visual symptoms)
- **Functional / non-organic visual loss** (diagnosis of exclusion)

Weakness

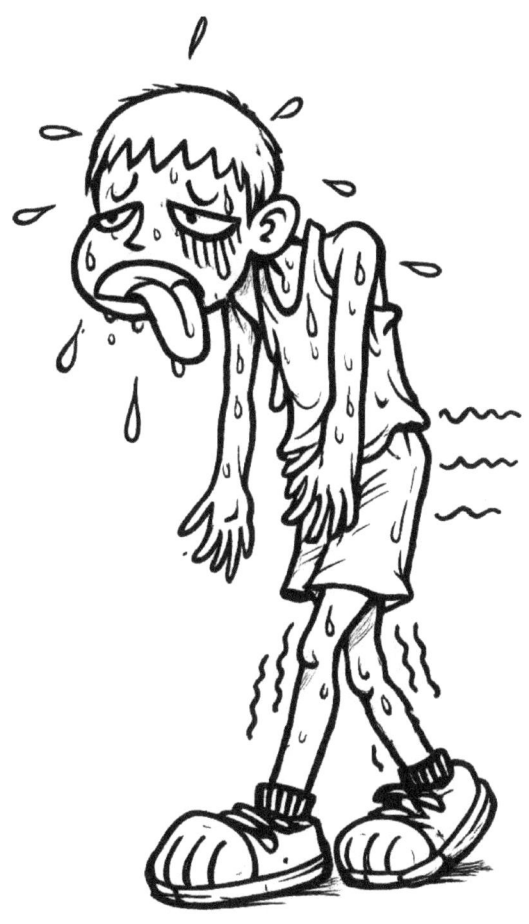

⚑ Red Flags: Weakness

- ⚠ Sudden onset focal weakness
- ⚠ Weakness with other focal neurological deficits
- ⚠ Weakness with back or neck pain, sensory level or sphincter disturbance
- ⚠ Rapidly progressive ascending weakness over hours to days
- ⚠ Weakness with bulbar or respiratory symptoms
- ⚠ Weakness in the context of fever, sepsis or meningism
- ⚠ Weakness with features of electrolyte or metabolic disturbance
- ⚠ Weakness in a patient with malignancy or on anticoagulation
- ⚠ Generalised proximal muscle weakness with myalgia or dark urine
- ⚠ Weakness with rash, arthralgia, weight loss or multisystem involvement

∏ Sudden onset focal weakness:

- ❖ **Implications/diagnoses:** Sudden onset focal weakness developing over seconds to minutes, especially if unilateral, strongly suggests an acute cerebrovascular event such as **ischaemic stroke**, **intracerebral haemorrhage** or **TIA**, with **TIA** considered if the deficit fully resolves quickly. This should be treated as **stroke** until proven otherwise because delayed recognition or treatment risks permanent neurological disability and loss of function.

- ❖ **Investigations:** Key investigations are urgent brain imaging with CT head, often combined with **CT angiography**, or **MRI brain** if available, together with a full **neurological examination**. Bedside assessments include **blood pressure, capillary glucose** and **ECG**, while blood tests such as **full blood count (FBC), urea and electrolytes (U&E), coagulation profile** and **lipid profile** help guide acute stroke management and secondary prevention. Immediate referral to the **stroke team** is essential so that suitability for **thrombolysis** or **thrombectomy** can be assessed.

∏ Weakness with other focal neurological deficits:

- ❖ **Implications/diagnoses:** Weakness accompanied by focal neurological features such as dysphasia, visual field loss, facial droop, hemisensory loss, neglect or ataxia indicates cortical or subcortical pathology. The main concerns are **ischaemic stroke, haemorrhagic stroke, TIA, primary brain tumour, brain metastases**, and sometimes **subdural haematoma** or other forms of **intracranial haemorrhage**.
- ❖ **Investigations:** This presentation should trigger cross-sectional imaging of the brain with **CT brain** or **MRI brain**, often with **vascular imaging** if **stroke** or a **vascular lesion** is suspected. A detailed **neurological examination** helps localise the lesion and prioritise imaging. Routine blood tests including **FBC, U&E, liver function tests (LFTs), coagulation profile** and **glucose** are performed to identify reversible contributors and to prepare for any potential interventions. Referral to **neurology** or **neurosurgery** is guided by imaging findings.

∏ **Weakness with back or neck pain, sensory level or sphincter disturbance:**
- ❖ **Implications/diagnoses:** Weakness associated with significant back or neck pain, a clear sensory level, saddle anaesthesia or new urinary retention or incontinence is highly suspicious for **spinal cord compression** or **cauda equina syndrome**. Causes include **disc prolapse, vertebral fracture, spinal metastases, epidural abscess or epidural haematoma**. These are neurosurgical emergencies because delay can result in permanent paralysis and irreversible bladder and bowel dysfunction.
- ❖ **Investigations:** Assessment should include a careful **neurological examination** documenting motor power, reflexes, tone, sensory level and perianal sensation. **Bladder scanning** to look for urinary retention is important, and inflammatory markers such as **FBC** and **ESR** or **CRP** may suggest infection or malignancy. The crucial investigation is urgent **MRI spine** of the relevant region to identify compressive lesions, followed by immediate discussion with **spinal surgery** or **neurosurgical** teams for definitive management.

∏ **Rapidly progressive ascending weakness over hours to days:**
- ❖ **Implications/diagnoses:** Rapidly progressive ascending weakness starting in the legs and moving proximally over hours to days, often with reduced or absent reflexes and distal tingling, is a classic red flag for **Guillain–Barré syndrome (GBS)** or related **acute inflammatory polyradiculoneuropathies**. The major dangers are **respiratory failure** and **autonomic instability**, which can develop even if limb weakness initially appears modest.

- ❖ **Investigations:** The priority is close monitoring of respiratory function with serial **vital capacity (VC)** or **forced vital capacity (FVC)** measurements, **peak flow** and **arterial or venous blood gases (ABG/VBG)**, along with frequent assessment of limb and cranial nerve strength. **Lumbar puncture (LP)** after the first few days may show **albumin cytologic dissociation** in the cerebrospinal fluid, and **nerve conduction studies (NCS)** or **electromyography (EMG)** help confirm the diagnosis. Baseline blood tests and **infection screening** are usually performed, and early **neurology** and **ICU** involvement is essential if respiratory compromise is anticipated.

∏ Weakness with bulbar or respiratory symptoms:

- ❖ **Implications/diagnoses:** Weakness that is accompanied by bulbar or respiratory features such as dysphagia, dysarthria, nasal speech, choking on fluids, orthopnoea or inability to speak full sentences suggests serious neuromuscular or brainstem pathology. Important diagnoses include **myasthenic crisis**, deterioration in **motor neurone disease (MND)**, **brainstem stroke** and other **neuromuscular junction disorders** such as **botulism**. These conditions pose an immediate threat to airway patency and ventilatory capacity.
- ❖ **Investigations:** Evaluation focuses first on respiratory reserve using measures such as **vital capacity (VC/FVC)**, **negative inspiratory force (NIF)** and **ABG/VBG**. A detailed **cranial nerve examination** is needed to identify **ptosis**, facial weakness, palatal involvement and fatigable weakness. If **brainstem stroke** is suspected, urgent **CT brain** or **MRI brain** is required. **Myasthenia gravis**–related tests such as **acetylcholine receptor (AChR) antibodies**, MuSK

antibodies and **electrophysiological studies (repetitive nerve stimulation / EMG)** can be arranged but must not delay supportive care or escalation to **intensive care (ICU)** if ventilation is at risk.

∏ Weakness in the context of fever, sepsis or meningism:

- ❖ **Implications/diagnoses:** Weakness occurring in a patient with fever, hypotension, tachycardia or meningism, including confusion, neck stiffness and photophobia, may reflect **sepsis** causing **encephalopathy** or **critical illness myopathy**. It can also be due to central nervous system infections such as **meningitis** or **encephalitis**, or **spinal epidural abscess** when severe back pain and neurological deficits coexist. These entities carry high morbidity and mortality if not rapidly addressed.
- ❖ **Investigations:** Management begins with a standard **sepsis work-up**, including **blood cultures, inflammatory markers (CRP, ESR), serum lactate, chest X-ray (CXR)** and **urinalysis with culture**. Where safe, **lumbar puncture (LP)** is performed to analyse **CSF** for **microscopy, culture** and **viral PCR** in suspected meningitis or encephalitis. If a **spinal epidural abscess** is suspected, urgent **MRI spine** is indicated. Empirical **intravenous antibiotics** are started according to local guidelines while investigations proceed, and ongoing monitoring of organ function with **U&E, LFTs** and **blood gases** is essential.

∏ Weakness with features of electrolyte or metabolic disturbance:

- ❖ **Implications/diagnoses:** Weakness accompanied by symptoms such as palpitations or arrhythmias, severe muscle cramps, gastrointestinal upset, polyuria, polydipsia or acute confusion suggests an underlying electrolyte or metabolic abnormality. Conditions of concern include **hypokalaemia, hyperkalaemia,** severe **hyponatraemia, hypernatremia, hypophosphatemia, hypocalcaemia, thyrotoxic periodic paralysis, adrenal crisis,** and decompensated diabetes such as **diabetic ketoacidosis (DKA)** or **hyperosmolar hyperglycaemic state (HHS)**. These can be rapidly life-threatening if not corrected.

- **Investigations:** Assessment requires urgent blood tests including **U&E, calcium, magnesium, phosphate, glucose** and **serum/urine ketones**, along with **ABG** or **VBG** to assess acid–base status and **lactate. Creatine** kinase **(CK)** should be checked if **rhabdomyolysis** is suspected. **Thyroid function tests (TFTs)** and **cortisol** or a **short Synacthen test** may be needed to evaluate endocrine causes. An **ECG** is crucial in suspected potassium abnormalities to detect conduction disturbances or arrhythmias and to guide immediate treatment.

∏ Weakness in a patient with malignancy or on anticoagulation:

- **Implications/diagnoses**

  New weakness in someone with known or suspected **malignancy**, or in a patient taking **anticoagulants** especially with recent trauma or headache, raises concern for **metastatic spinal cord compression, brain metastases** or **intracranial** or **spinal haematoma** such as **subdural haematoma** or **epidural haematoma**. Failure to act quickly can result in irreversible neurological deficits, including paraplegia, cognitive impairment or seizures.

- **Investigations:** Urgent **MRI spine** is the investigation of choice for suspected **metastatic cord compression**, while **MRI brain** or **CT head** is used to identify **brain metastases** or **intracranial haemorrhage**. **CT head** is often the initial test for suspected **subdural haematoma** in an anticoagulated or head-injured patient. Additional tests include **coagulation profile (INR, PT, APTT)**, drug levels where relevant, and baseline blood tests such as **FBC** and **U&E**, with rapid involvement of **oncology**, **neurology** and **neurosurgery** to plan **steroids**, **radiotherapy**, **surgery** or **reversal** of **anticoagulation**.

∏ Generalised proximal muscle weakness with myalgia or dark urine:

- ❖ **Implications/diagnoses:** Generalised proximal muscle weakness, especially difficulty climbing stairs, rising from a chair or lifting the arms, combined with muscle pain or dark, cola-coloured urine, suggests an underlying myopathic process. Important causes include **inflammatory myopathies** such as **polymyositis** and **dermatomyositis**, **endocrine myopathies** related to **thyroid disease** or **Cushing's syndrome**, and **rhabdomyolysis** triggered by **statins**, **alcohol**, **prolonged seizures**, **toxins** or **crush injuries**. These can lead to **acute kidney injury (AKI)** if muscle breakdown is severe.

- ❖ **Investigations:** Core investigations include measurement of **creatine kinase (CK)**, which is often markedly elevated in **rhabdomyolysis**, and assessment of renal function with **U&E** and **serum creatinine**. **Urinalysis** is used to detect **myoglobinuria**, and **LFTs** can show secondary abnormalities. **Thyroid function tests (TFTs)** and **cortisol** levels help identify endocrine causes. **Autoimmune screening** with **ANA** and **myositis-specific antibodies**, along with **EMG** and **muscle biopsy** arranged through **neurology** or **rheumatology**, further defines the underlying myopathy.

∏ Weakness with rash, arthralgia, weight loss or multisystem involvement:

- ❖ **Implications/diagnoses:** Weakness occurring alongside rash, arthralgia, constitutional symptoms such as weight loss, fevers or night sweats, and evidence of multi-organ involvement suggests **systemic vasculitis, connective tissue disease** such as **systemic lupus erythematosus (SLE)**, or a **paraneoplastic syndrome**. These conditions can affect muscle, peripheral nerves, kidneys, lungs and other organs, leading to significant morbidity if not detected and treated early.

- ❖ **Investigations:** The investigative approach includes **FBC**, **ESR** and **CRP** to assess systemic inflammation, together with **U&E** and **LFTs**. **Urinalysis** is important to detect **haematuria** or **proteinuria** that may signify renal involvement. **Autoantibody panels** such as **ANA**, **ENA**, **ANCA** and **complement levels** help narrow down specific rheumatological diagnoses, and **CK** is measured if muscle involvement is suspected. Cross-sectional imaging such as **CT chest/abdomen/pelvis** may be needed to look for underlying **malignancy**, with **rheumatology** or **oncology** input depending on the clinical scenario.

🗝 Key Points:

For limb weakness, think **FAST & FOCUSED** – you're trying to answer: *where is the lesion, how urgent is it, and what's the likely cause?*

- ❖ **First question:** *Is this an emergency?* – RED FLAGS

Treat these as **time-critical**:

- Sudden onset weakness (seconds–minutes) ± face/speech problems
    → think **stroke/TIA** – urgent stroke pathway.

- **Rapidly progressive ascending weakness, areflexia, difficulty walking, breathlessness**

  → think **Guillain–Barré** / acute neuropathy – urgent admission, monitor vital capacity.

- **Weak legs + severe back pain + saddle anaesthesia, urinary retention or incontinence**

  → **Cauda equina** – emergency MRI spine + neurosurgery.

- **Neck/back pain + bilateral weakness or sensory level, brisk reflexes**

  → **Spinal cord compression** – urgent MRI, steroids as per local protocol.

- **Weakness with ptosis, diplopia, bulbar symptoms (dysarthria, dysphagia) or fatigability**

  → **Myasthenic crisis** risk – monitor respiratory function, consider ICU.

- **Weakness + dyspnoea, chest pain, palpitations**

  → consider **hyperkalaemia**, arrhythmia, myopathy, PE, sepsis.

- If any of these are present → **senior review and urgent investigations immediately.**

❖ Clarify the pattern – *localise the lesion*

Key axes:

- **Onset & time course**
  - Sudden → vascular
  - Subacute days–weeks → inflammatory/infective
  - Chronic months–years → degenerative, hereditary, metabolic

- **Distribution**
    - **Hemiparesis (face + arm ± leg)** → brain (stroke, tumour)
    - **Paraparesis (both legs)** → spinal cord (cord compression, myelopathy)
    - **Quadriparesis (all limbs)** → high cord, brainstem, or generalised disease
    - **Distal > proximal** → neuropathy (e.g. diabetes)
    - **Proximal > distal** → myopathy, neuromuscular junction (e.g. myasthenia)
- **UMN vs LMN signs**
    - **UMN:** increased tone, brisk reflexes, upgoing plantar
    - **LMN:** wasting, fasciculations, reduced tone, absent reflexes
- **Focused history – a few essentials**
- **Exact onset:** date/time, sudden vs gradual, stepwise vs relapsing/remitting.
- **Preceding events:** infection, vaccination, trauma, surgery, new drugs (statins, steroids).
- **Associated symptoms:**
    - Sensory change, pain, back/neck pain
    - Visual, speech, swallowing, facial symptoms
    - Bladder/bowel changes
    - Fatigue, weight loss, systemic features
- **Past history:** stroke, diabetes, cancer, autoimmune disease.
- **Functional impact:** walking, stairs, transfers, falls.

Focused examination – what you must check

- **Vital signs** (incl. sats) – look for sepsis, hypoxia, arrhythmias.
- **Cranial nerves** – face, speech, swallowing, eye movements, visual fields.
- **Tone, power, reflexes, plantar responses** – both sides.
- **Sensory exam** – light touch, pin, vibration, proprioception; look for a sensory level.
- **Gait & coordination** if safe – ataxia, foot drop, spastic gait.
- **Spine/back exam** – tenderness, deformity.
- **Respiratory effort** if neuromuscular disease suspected – count to 20 in one breath, look for use of accessory muscles.

Initial investigations (typical acute take)

- **Bloods:** FBC, U&E, LFT, CRP, ESR, CK, glucose, bone profile, B12/folate, TFTs as needed.
- **Urgent CT head ± CT angiography** if stroke suspected.
- **MRI brain/spine** if cord compression, demyelination, tumour, etc. suspected.
- **ECG** ± troponin if cardiac cause possible.
- **CXR** if infection, malignancy, neuromuscular weakness.
- **Further tests** guided by findings: LP, nerve conduction studies/EMG, autoimmune/myopathy panels, etc.

Simple mental framework (for exams & ward rounds)

Use **"VINDICATE"** for causes of limb weakness:

- **V**ascular – stroke, spinal infarct
- **I**nfective/Inflammatory – abscess, myelitis, GBS, myositis
- **N**eoplastic – primary/secondary CNS or spinal tumours
- **D**egenerative – MND, MS, myopathies
- **I**atrogenic – drugs (steroids, statins), post-op
- **C**ongenital – muscular dystrophies, hereditary neuropathies
- **A**utoimmune – myasthenia, CIDP, vasculitis
- **T**raumatic – cord injury, nerve palsy
- **E**ndocrine/Metabolic – thyroid, Cushing's, electrolyte disorders, B12

ABC approach to weakness (evaluation + workup):

A — Assessment and immediate threats

- **ABCs + vitals + capillary glucose** (hypoglycaemia can mimic neuro deficit)
- **Clarify severity now**
  - **Airway/ventilation risk:** bulbar symptoms (dysarthria, dysphagia), weak cough, pooling secretions
  - **Breathing:** tachypnoea, use of accessory muscles, paradoxical breathing
- **Time-critical "can't miss" causes**
  - **Stroke/TIA/ICH:** sudden focal weakness ± speech/vision changes
  - **Spinal cord compression / cauda equina:** bilateral leg weakness, saddle anaesthesia, bladder/bowel dysfunction

- **Guillain–Barré (GBS):** progressive ascending weakness, areflexia, autonomic instability
- **Myasthenic crisis:** fatigable weakness + bulbar/respiratory involvement
- **Severe electrolyte disorders:** K+, Ca/Mg, phosphate (periodic paralysis)
- **Sepsis/meningitis/encephalitis:** weakness with fever, confusion
- **Rhabdomyolysis:** myalgia + dark urine + weakness

- **Immediate actions**
  - **If stroke suspected:** activate stroke pathway (time of onset/last known well)
  - **If cord/cauda signs:** urgent MRI spine + neurosurgical/ortho referral; treat suspected malignant compression urgently per protocol
  - **If respiratory/bulbar weakness:** sit upright, oxygen if needed, urgent senior/ITU review; consider early NIV/intubation
  - **If severe hyper/hypokalaemia or hypoglycaemia:** treat immediately
  - **If suspected GBS/MG crisis:** urgent neuro/ICU input; monitor respiratory function closely

B — Bedside assessment (focused history & exam)

Focused history (key discriminators)

- **Onset & tempo**
  - **Sudden** (seconds–minutes): stroke/ICH, seizure (Todd's paresis)
  - **Hours–days:** GBS, myelitis, infection, toxic/metabolic

- - **Weeks–months:** malignancy, motor neuron disease, myopathy, neuropathy
- **Distribution/pattern**
  - **Unilateral:** stroke, cortical lesion
  - **Bilateral legs:** cord lesion, GBS
  - **Proximal > distal:** myopathy (steroids, inflammatory myositis)
  - **Distal > proximal:** neuropathy
  - **Fluctuating/fatigable:** myasthenia gravis
- **Associated symptoms**
  - **Speech/face:** dysphasia, facial droop (stroke)
  - **Sensory level/back pain:** cord compression/myelopathy
  - **Bladder/bowel/saddle anaesthesia:** cauda equina
  - **Diplopia/ptosis:** MG, brainstem pathology
  - **Painful weakness:** radiculopathy, myositis, rhabdo
  - **Recent infection/vaccine:** GBS
  - **Systemic:** fever, weight loss, night sweats (infection/malignancy)
- **Medication/toxin**
  - Statins (myopathy/rhabdo), steroids (myopathy), alcohol, cocaine
  - Diuretics/laxatives (K+ disturbance), chemo (neuropathy)
- **PMH**
  - Diabetes (neuropathy), thyroid disease, autoimmune, cancer, AF

Focused examination (localise: brain vs cord vs peripheral nerve vs NMJ vs muscle)

- **General**
  - Mental state, speech, cranial nerves (face, eye movements, bulbar function)
- **Motor**
  - Tone (spastic vs flaccid), power pattern, pronator drift
- **Reflexes**
  - **Hyperreflexia/clonus/Babinski** → UMN (brain/cord)
  - **Hyporeflexia/areflexia** → LMN/peripheral/GBS
- **Sensation**
  - Dermatomal loss, **sensory level**, vibration/proprioception
- **Coordination & gait**
  - Ataxia, Romberg; gait if safe
- **NMJ signs**
  - Fatigability, ptosis, Cogan lid twitch; count aloud to assess bulbar fatigue
- **Respiratory bedside tests (if concern)**
  - **FVC, NIF** (or single breath count) + ABG/VBG if ventilatory failure suspected

C- Core investigations (workup)

- **Bedside / immediate**
  - **Capillary glucose**
  - **ECG** (K+ abnormalities, arrhythmia/AF)
  - **Urinalysis** (blood without RBCs → rhabdo)

- **Bloods (baseline)**
  - **FBC, CRP**
  - **U&Es + K+, Ca, Mg, PO4**
  - **LFTs**
  - **CK** (myopathy/rhabdo)
  - **TSH**
  - **B12/folate**
  - **HbA1c** (if neuropathy pattern/unknown DM)
- **Targeted tests (based on pattern)**
  - **Stroke:** urgent CT head ± CTA/MRI per pathway; glucose, coagulation, troponin often included locally
  - **Cord/cauda: MRI spine** (urgent)
  - **GBS:** lumbar puncture (albuminocytologic dissociation—often later), NCS/EMG; monitor FVC closely
  - **MG:** AChR/MuSK antibodies, bedside fatigability tests; consider neurophysiology; ABG if crisis
  - **Inflammatory myopathy:** ESR/CRP, myositis panel, consider MRI muscle
  - **Infection/encephalitis:** blood cultures, LP, brain imaging as indicated
- **When to escalate to specialist tests**
  - **EMG/NCS** (neuropathy/GBS/MND/NMJ)
  - **MRI brain** (atypical neuro signs, demyelination, brainstem/cerebellar features)
- **UMN (Brain/Spinal cord) weakness**
  - **Pattern:** pyramidal distribution (arm extensors + leg flexors weaker), often **unilateral** (brain) or **bilateral legs** (cord)
  - **Tone:** ↑ tone/spasticity

- **Reflexes:** ↑ **reflexes**, clonus
- **Plantar: upgoing (Babinski)**
- **Other clues:** sensory level (cord), aphasia/neglect/ visual field defect (brain)

- **LMN (Anterior horn / root / peripheral nerve) weakness**
  - **Pattern: focal** (root/nerve) or distal symmetric (polyneuropathy)
  - **Tone:** ↓ **tone/flaccid**
  - **Reflexes:** ↓**/absent reflexes**
  - **Other clues: fasciculations**, muscle wasting, neuropathic pain/paresthesia
  - **Sensory:** often present in peripheral neuropathy; **radicular** sensory loss in roots

- **Neuromuscular junction (NMJ) weakness**
  - **Pattern: fatigable**, fluctuating; ocular/bulbar common
  - **Tone/reflexes:** usually **normal**
  - **Sensation: normal**
  - **Clues: ptosis**, diplopia, dysarthria/dysphagia, worse later in day; improves with rest
  - **Crisis red flags:** weak cough, pooling secretions, low FVC/NIF

- **Muscle (Myopathy) weakness**
  - **Pattern: proximal > distal** (difficulty rising from chair, climbing stairs, lifting arms)
  - **Tone:** normal or ↓
  - **Reflexes:** preserved until late (may be reduced if severe)
  - **Sensation: normal**

- **Clues:** myalgia/tenderness; **CK often ↑** (inflammatory/rhabdo), rash (dermatomyositis); steroid/statin history
- **"Top localisers" at the bedside**
  - **Face/arm/leg + speech/vision** → brain (stroke pathway)
  - **Both legs + sensory level/back pain + bladder/bowel** → cord/cauda (urgent MRI)
  - **Ascending weakness + areflexia** → GBS (monitor FVC/autonomics)
  - **Ocular/bulbar + fatigability** → MG (watch for crisis)
  - **Proximal weakness + high CK/myalgia** → myopathy/rhabdo

Red flags for weakness - "WEAKNESS"

W – Was fine, now weak (sudden onset)

- Sudden limb weakness over **seconds–minutes** → **stroke / intracranial bleed**.

E – Evolving fast

- Weakness **worsening over hours–days**, especially ascending → **GBS, myelitis, cord compression**.

A – Autonomic changes

- **Urinary retention, incontinence, saddle anaesthesia → cauda equina / cord compression.**

K – Knife-like back or neck pain

- Severe new **back/neck pain** ± bilateral weakness/sensory level → **spinal cord / epidural lesion**.

N – Not able to walk

- New inability to **stand or mobilise** → significant **cord, stroke, or neuromuscular disease**.

E – Evil history

- **Cancer, weight loss, immunosuppression, recent infection → metastatic cord compression, abscess, paraneoplastic, GBS.**

S – Short of breath or swallowing difficulty

- **Dyspnoea, weak cough, dysphagia, dysarthria, ptosis, diplopia → myasthenic crisis, GBS, brainstem stroke.**

S – Stroke signs

- Weakness plus **facial droop**, **speech or visual disturbance** → treat as **stroke** until proven otherwise.

www.ingramcontent.com/pod-product-compliance
Ingram Content Group UK Ltd.
Pitfield, Milton Keynes, MK11 3LW, UK
UKHW061223180426
11947UKWH00027B/1984